Cholesterol is Not the Culprit

A Guide to Preventing Heart Disease

D0517999

Fred A. Kummerow, Ph.D.

with Jean M. Kummerow, Ph.D.

Published February, 2014 by Spacedoc Media, LLC

Copyright © 2014

ISBN: 978-0-9833835-6-7

This is a newly updated edition of
a book previously published as:
*Cholesterol Won't Kill You But Trans Fat Could
Separating Scientific Fact from Nutritional Fiction*

Cover image: Yusuf Yilmaz/Shutterstock.com

The opinions expressed in this book are for information and education purposes only and should not be used to diagnose or treat any illness, disease, or other medical condition.

Always consult with a qualified medical professional before making medication, diet, dietary supplement, exercise, or lifestyle changes or decisions.

Contents

Introduction

There are thousands of books on diet and nutrition full of advice on what to eat to live longer and healthier. Yet that advice seems to be constantly changing and even conflicting, and thus ends up being continually confusing. This is in part due to the fact that the human body is very complex—there are over 23,000 chemical processes in a human being.[1] Some nutritional guidance pays attention to one process but forgets the chemistry involved and the impact on the whole body. Other advice is based on outdated research or even worse, is not based in science at all, and is, in actuality, a myth.

For example, for decades the nutritional advice was to eat margarine and avoid butter because it contained cholesterol, and cholesterol has unfairly been seen as "bad." Both margarine and butter contain something called trans fat and those trans fats were assumed to be the same and thus work the same way in the body, although that is not the case. This was never the advice in my own household since I knew the chemistry of both foods and that the actual research supported the opposite! Now the popular advice (and government regulations) have caught up to the basic research and are saying that because margarines contain manufactured trans fat that works differently (actually negatively) in the body than the natural trans fat of butter, it should be avoided. Butter is better. More on this issue later.

You will find this book focuses on the basic chemistry of food; this includes cholesterol and trans fat, how the body works, and how food fits into that chemistry. We will explain the key processes in the body and why food is so important to its function. Much of the "why" comes from basic information about how the chemistry of the body works. This book explains the chemistry of some of those basic processes and how cholesterol is part of that process. We'll also look at the chemistry of trans fat to help you understand why eating it does not keep your heart healthy.

You'll find us returning again and again to the basics of a healthy diet:

- Protein from sources such as grains, milk, eggs, meat, and fish
- Energy sources from carbohydrates and sugar
- Fat from animal and vegetable products
- Fiber from grains, fruits, and vegetables
- Minerals from protein sources, grains, fruits, and vegetables
- Vitamins from protein sources, grains, fruits, and vegetables
- Liquids

These ingredients come together in different ways through chemistry to provide us with energy and with what we need to continue to build cells throughout our lifetime. They are used in a delicate balance, and anything upsetting that balance has negative consequences for our health.

Because I have spoken the language of science for so long, I find it difficult to translate my knowledge and understanding into laypeople's language. My daughter, Jean, a psychologist and an author, stepped in to help with that part. She kept at me to explain and then explain again the complexities of the science. At times, even she had to give up and let some of the "pure" science remain. You may not understand all of the science but it is the only way to explain the complex interactions of diet and body chemistry. We've tried to summarize and translate the research findings cited so that you can understand the studies, what they mean, and how they help us determine what to eat. Just note the numerical citation that leads to the references and the original study and look it up. You may notice some of the same nutritional topics discussed in several chapters because those topics are important to several aspects of our body's use of food, and we do not expect you to remember all of the background from one chapter to the next. It can be even more difficult to eat only healthy foods when so much unhealthy food is available in fast food outlets and restaurants as well as our own kitchen.

You will find a lot in this book related to diet and heart disease; it is the number one cause of death in the U.S. and throughout much of the world and also the focus of the majority of my career. To me, researching diet and heart disease is like being the detective in a good mystery book who follows clue after clue and finally comes up with an unexpected answer. The detective is always trying to find out who and what killed the person. For example, over 100 years ago, scientific detectives found that single cells (like bacteria) could invade a human being and cause death. Since then, detectives have been identifying more and more scientific reasons for causes of death, and in the process identifying the scientific processes of living. One of these processes involves cholesterol, which actually makes life possible. Some detectives view cholesterol as the killer in heart disease, but I'll show you why that's not so. Thinking that cholesterol is the killer is quite different than thinking that cholesterol is a clue to the killer, and I hope you'll agree with that latter conclusion. In this book you will read about new clues for the heart disease detective and what I believe is/are really the killer(s) in heart disease. Some of the clues focus on the biochemistry of the diet in heart disease.[2] Other clues lead to what you can do to improve your diet and prevent heart disease. One of these, for example, is to eliminate trans fat from your diet. As we'll explain later, trans fat interferes with blood flow, which can result in sudden death. And some of the clues also take you into yet another story by including possible government action to help make all of us healthier.

My own eating recommendations are in the last chapter. Those recommendations are for readily available foods, not exotic combinations available only in health food stores or from organic farms. Most of the foods for good nutrition are available in the outside ring of a typical supermarket; many of the foods that are less nutritious are on the inside aisles. It can be difficult to grocery shop for only healthy foods even when you are motivated to do so. It can be even more difficult to eat only healthy foods when so much unhealthy food is available in fast food outlets and restaurants as well as our own kitchens.

We hope in reading this book, you'll not only learn what is healthy to eat, but also why it is healthy to do so. How the body uses food to make what we need to keep going is an incredible, almost magical, process. We—as well as all animals and plants—are not programmed to live forever, but we can certainly increase the number of high quality years of life. Eating well (that is eating foods with high nutritional value) in moderation may help us all do so.

CHAPTER 1: Why the Concern About Cholesterol?

If you read a newspaper, surf the internet, listen to television ads, and/or take the advice of most physicians, you would think cholesterol is bad and should be cut out of the diet because of its link to heart disease. This leaves the wrong impression about cholesterol. Did you know that:

- Cholesterol is necessary for every cell of the human body to exist, and without cholesterol, human beings could not exist.

- People make their own cholesterol because their bodies need it to live. A typical adult male naturally makes about 900 milligrams (mg) of cholesterol in his liver each day unless that cholesterol is obtained in his diet.

- A typical diet now contains approximately 400 mg of cholesterol.

- Most foods that contain cholesterol also are the greatest sources of protein, such as eggs, dairy, and meat products.

- It is protein that carries cholesterol successfully through the arteries and veins in the body and allows for its appropriate use. If protein sources are cut from the diet because of concern about their cholesterol content, we are actually creating more, not fewer problems since protein must perform not only a cholesterol-carrying function, but also serve as building blocks for cells (and we are made up of 50,000 trillion cells).[1,2]

- An egg, when eaten with a fiber-containing food, like whole wheat bread, does not add significantly to a person's blood cholesterol level, even though one egg itself contains 210-220 mg of cholesterol (see chapter 3).

Cholesterol has been viewed in a variety of ways in the past. In 1963, for example, some of these were summarized: "Our attitude toward cholesterol is best exemplified by an outline of the recent history of its public relations:[3]

- 1947: cholesterol found to be associated with atherosclerosis;
- 1950: cholesterol is killing you;
- 1954: cholesterol, stress, and lack of exercise are killing you;
- 1962: cholesterol is not helping other things kill you;
- 1963: anything that helps make sex hormones (from cholesterol) cannot be all bad;
- [The future prediction:] Cholesterol is a good guy."

Well, we are not yet at the place where cholesterol is considered the good guy but perhaps we'll get there yet. It took decades to get to the point where people saw trans fat as "bad," and it will likely take decades before people see cholesterol as "good." This chapter discusses the positive aspects of cholesterol, why you need it, and how you can get it in the right amounts. It also reviews how cholesterol came to be implicated in the heart disease mystery, including what heart disease is. We'll discuss what we do know about diet and heart disease, and what you can do now to help improve your diet in light of the research.

What is Cholesterol?
Since the word "cholesterol" is so prevalent in the discussion of diet and heart disease, we need to first understand what it really is and its purpose in our bodies. Before cholesterol existed in cells there could only be one-cell organisms.[4] These organisms contained only a

protective membrane composed of phospholipids (a type of lipid that forms the protective layer around the cell), a compound that could not prevent the entry of salt into the cell. As the oceans became saltier, cells could not survive. A protective factor might have become available from plant tissue. A molecule named Brassinosteroid (which has a structure almost identical to cholesterol) could have incorporated into the membrane to protect the cell against the elements. Brassinosteroid is still present at low concentrations throughout the plant kingdom today.[5] This cholesterol-containing organism became so successful that it formed clumps of cells and developed a circulation system, like arteries and veins, to supply nutrients. These clumps developed into sea life and eventually animal life on land. The argument about when human life began should be directly linked to when cholesterol began to be part of an organism's cell membrane that made human life possible.

We humans are born with cholesterol already surrounded by a phospholipid membrane to protect our cells, and with the ability to make more of it in our liver. Cholesterol is essential for all animal life, but not as a nutrient or source of food. Without cholesterol our bodies couldn't replace cells when needed so that we can keep on living. Cholesterol is encased by a phospholipid membrane for every one of the 50,000 trillion cells in the body, so a lot of cholesterol is required.[2] Cholesterol is a good and necessary compound, not a bad one. In actuality, without cholesterol we would not exist.

Essentially, cholesterol is a waxy-like substance produced by the liver for our bodies to use in our daily living. It is a chemical that is insoluble in water, meaning it doesn't dissolve in water, and thus is available to construct a membrane around a cell that sheds water and consequently protects it. Every one of our 50,000 trillion cells "floats" in a lymph fluid, which is composed of 98% water. This fluid contains the salts of sodium, potassium, calcium, and magnesium as well as nutrients from the blood for transfer into the cell. Without the protective mantle of membranes, the salts in the life-sustaining fluid that surrounds each cell could diffuse (enter) through the cell wall and kill the cell.[4] Those salts have their own purposes in the body, which we will explain in a later chapter.

Cholesterol in our blood helps cells replace themselves and protects the working elements in the cells. These working elements are the parts that (a) convert food into energy, (b) contain the nucleus, which is how the cell reproduces itself, and (c) manufacture protein and other elements needed by the cell.[2] All animals, including humans, have and require each of their cells to be encased by a cholesterol-containing membrane. Thus experiments on the effects of cholesterol in the diet can be conducted on animals such as swine, chickens, and rats, instead of on human beings[3].

The French chemist Michel Chevreul first identified cholesterol in 1815 by differentiating it from other wax-like compounds.[6] He named the substance cholesterine, which comes from chole and stereos (Greek for bile and solid, respectively). After additional study of its chemical composition, another component of the substance called a hydroxyl group was discovered, and the name changed to cholesterol to make the name more accurate.

How is Cholesterol Carried in our Bodies?

Although scientists knew about the substances like phospholipids, cholesterol and fats (or fatty acids), they did not know how these could be made in the body until over a century later. Two Nobel Prizes for medicine were awarded to researchers who figured out how fatty acids and cholesterol were used and made in the body. In 1953, Hans Krebs received a Nobel Prize for discovering the first part of the mystery—how fatty acids are used in a pathway now called the Krebs Cycle.[7] Later Konrad Bloch's discovery of

10

how cholesterol is made from acetyl CoA won the Nobel Prize in 1964.[8]

To clarify at least part of this prize-winning research, here's a simplified explanation. All of what we eat gets "chopped" up by enzymes into very small chemical fragments (called acetyl CoA) which serve as a source of energy as well as a source of building blocks for our cells to be put together in different ways.

A "healthy" diet provides the necessary blocks for a healthy body. An "unhealthy" diet can provide energy, but not all of the right building blocks and eventually people will suffer ill health from this lack. A building can look good for a short period of time, but will fall down if shoddy construction materials are used. It's the same with our bodies; the right foods need to be in our bodies in the right amounts so that the right building blocks get made. The wrong amounts of food (too much fat or sugar, for example) furnish only energy, but have to go somewhere if the energy boost is not needed. This excessive fat or sugar likely ends up as more fat deposited on the person's body and in the arteries, the beginning of heart disease. Some of those nutrient building blocks have dual roles—to carry food as well as serve as the nutrient itself. For example, the fat that is absorbed through the intestines cannot float on its own in the blood, but rather combines with a protein (albumin) for its ride through the blood, so to speak. The cholesterol that is also absorbed from food in the intestine rides through the blood on a lipoprotein, a combination of fat and protein. Protein, as you can see, must be part of the building blocks since they "carry" both fat and cholesterol in the blood.

Each cell in the body has its own composition (e.g., cells in the eyes have a different composition than those in the brain), but they are all made by the same mechanism that has been operating the same way in microorganisms for over two billion years before humans arrived on earth.[2] This metabolic process involves taking the nutrients, sugar, fat, and protein out of the blood, and using enzymes to convert these nutrients into energy as well as building blocks.[9] Each cell has a component named the mitochondria which converts fat and sugar to the energy that is needed to keep the cell "alive" and another component named the endoplasmic reticulum that makes protein, fat, and sugar into building blocks that are used to construct the cell itself. The endoplasmic reticulum needs two essential fatty acids (linoleic and linolenic acid) and eight essential amino acids that it cannot make itself, but are present in the complete protein in eggs, milk, and meat. The cell uses an essential component in every living cell whether a single cell like a bacteria or as a complex of cells like a human being. This component is called acetyl CoA, a two-carbon component as simple as the two-carbon component in vinegar. Acetyl CoA serves as a source of energy and is also used by the enzymes in the cell to construct a component as complex as cholesterol. The necessary cell components that are synthesized in the endoplasmic reticulum are transferred to the golgi complex (another component in the cell) for their distribution in the cell. Each cell in the body works identically to provide energy and structural components that make it possible to repair itself and build new cells. Normally, all of the essential components end up in the cell where they are used for building body cells or adipose (fat) cells. The fat in albumin and the cholesterol in lipoproteins in the blood that are not used up in the normal way may end up being made into debris (atherosclerosis) in the arterial wall, an abnormal use. The abnormal use means that first, fatty streaks appear in the arteries, followed by plaques (atherosclerosis),[10] as explained later in this chapter.

How Much Cholesterol is Made in our Bodies?

Knowing how much cholesterol is naturally made in our bodies also helps us to understand more about cholesterol. One study showed that 840-910 mg[11], and another 367-1407 mg[12], of cholesterol are made from acetyl CoA in the liver during a 24 hour period. This means each day that amount of cholesterol needs to be produced by the liver or furnished through food sources for normal cell functioning. If you eat foods containing cholesterol, your liver makes less cholesterol. One study[12] showed that only 34-63% of dietary cholesterol is absorbed through the intestinal tract, and probably less if you eat lots of fiber. Your body has a mechanism that stops the making of cholesterol in the liver so as to regulate the amount in the blood each day.[13, 14] This ensures that you have enough, but not too much, cholesterol for your body to use.

What Is Heart Disease?

Before proceeding with looking at cholesterol and heart disease, we need to take a step back and understand more about the heart and heart disease. The heart is a hollow, muscular organ composed of four chambers that work together to pump 13,000 liters (more than 13,700 quarts) of blood throughout itself and the body every 24 hours.[15] The heart is supplied with nutrients and oxygen-rich blood through a series of coronary arteries. The word "coronary" means crown, and the arteries that circle the heart appear like a crown.

Since the heart is a muscle, you can deliberately exercise it to increase its capacity. First you create a baseline of your normal resting pulse rate by counting the beats for 15 seconds and multiplying by four. Next do some type of vigorous activity, the type of which depends on your physical condition. For some people, walking is vigorous while for others, it is running or boxing. Check your pulse after a few minutes of that activity and monitor it until it comes back down to your baseline level. If you continue that program for several weeks, you will notice that the time it takes for your pulse to return to baseline lessens indicating that your heart muscle has gotten stronger.

Heart disease is usually referred to as Coronary Heart Disease (CHD). It is a multi-factorial disease, meaning many factors contribute to its occurrence. These include genetics, age, smoking, and diet including fat intake, cholesterol metabolism, and cell structure. Research on heart disease is a worldwide activity, although little *basic* research on the chemical processes involved in heart disease is being carried out today[16]. Heart disease is the major cause of death throughout the world, especially now that the average life expectancy is longer. It has been documented as a cause of death for centuries but it wasn't until the 1920s that the major cause of deaths from heart disease was identified as coronary artery blockage, *and* not a problem with the heart itself.[17] Pathologists have examined thousands of human aortas (the large artery leaving the heart) from various population groups.[10] They found that some aortas contained only small areas of lipid (fat) deposits and others contained "debris" called "plaques" that hinder the flow of blood.[10] Why the small areas of lipid deposits called fatty streaks in the aorta of some people do not develop into "plaques" has been under study since 1950.

There are two ways heart disease leads to blockages and perhaps death—the slower process of atherosclerosis and the sudden one of an "unexpected" heart attack. The first way, atherosclerosis, is a condition in the coronary arteries that leads to heart disease.[9] It involves the gradual change in composition of the arteries eventually leading to blockage of the coronary artery so that no blood gets to the heart. "Debris" made up of calcium, accumulates in the intimal wall (the first layer) of the coronary artery. The first place the debris accumulates is at the branches of the arteries. Dr. M.E. DeBakey, a pioneer in cardiac bypass surgery, found that more debris accumulates at those branches.[18,19] Think of a river and its tributaries or branches; debris is much more likely to accumulate at the branches than in the free flowing river.[20] The arteries get narrower and narrower over time and less and less blood flows through the coronary arteries. It is impossible at present to completely avoid the build up of debris. Some of the debris such as trans fat incorporates into the arterial cell itself and changes its composition and function.[21-23] With age, eventually all the arterial cells themselves change in composition, decreasing the blood flow and leading to heart disease.[22] This change occurs in both the arteries that "feed" the heart, and the peripheral arteries that "feed" the rest of the body. The trick is to delay that change as long as possible by, for example, cutting out fried foods.

The second type of heart disease is more sudden and was not prevalent in the U.S. before 1920.[22] It involves the way blood flows and the lack of a key chemical to keep the blood flowing (prostacyclin) with an "overdose" of a chemical that clots the blood (thromboxane). Both of these processes are affected by the type of fats in our bodies. Manufactured trans fat plays a major role leading to heart disease since it interferes with the natural blood flow processes. More on this later.

How Cholesterol Became a Health Marker (And its Limitations)

Now back to cholesterol and the heart disease mystery. The hypothesis that high cholesterol is the major risk factor in heart disease was first based on a study in 1906 by a Russian professor of pathology named Nikolai Anitschkow.[24] He fed rabbits cholesterol-containing diets. He then noticed that these rabbits had atherosclerosis in their coronary arteries that resembled the atherosclerosis in human coronary arteries; the arteries of rabbits looked just like the arteries of people who had died of heart disease. This original Russian study implicated cholesterol in heart disease. Anitschkow also fed the same diet to rats and noticed that they did not develop atherosclerosis. However, the results of this rat study were ignored. Researchers and

15

physicians interpreted his rabbit cholesterol study to mean that restricting cholesterol-containing food from the food supply, such as eggs, meat, and milk, may prevent coronary heart disease. In looking further at this study, it is important to note the problem with the animal chosen for the experiment.

Decades later, with additional scientific techniques, this study was repeated with rabbits and rats.[25] Rabbits have no cholesterol in their diet in the first place. Since their livers manufactured all the cholesterol that their cells needed, they did not need to develop a way of handling the excess cholesterol they ingested in the experiments. Consequently the rabbits were doomed to end up with atherosclerosis because the cholesterol from their "unnatural" diet accumulated in their body and could not be handled. The excess cholesterol needed someplace to go, so it eventually ended up first in the liver and then in the arteries. In rats, excess cholesterol also ended up in the liver. However, unlike rabbits, rats have two antioxidant enzymes that could handle the cholesterol accumulation. An enzyme is a molecule that facilitates reactions. Antioxidant enzymes in particular are used by the liver to break down oxidized material. Rats, thus, did not develop the atherosclerosis that the rabbits did. However, with much greater amounts of dietary cholesterol, rats also could not handle cholesterol.

Before World War II (1940 - 1945), little was known about how cholesterol and fat were used by the body. This was evident in badly wounded soldiers who needed more calories to recover than the calories from glucose (sugar) provided by intravenous infusion into their veins. Research programs were begun to find a way to add fat for intravenous use. The Army Medical Corps therefore granted contracts to medical schools for the development of a satisfactory way to add the fat for intravenous use. Dr. Larry Hursh (deceased), who later became director of the University of Illinois student hospital, was medical director of this research program. He told me that none of the medical schools were able to come up with a satisfactory way of introducing fat directly into the vein. Three years after the war, the US congress established the National Institutes of Health (NIH), which funded a medical school to find out the answers as to why fat and cholesterol could not be introduced into the veins by intravenous infusion. It was shown by a group of researchers at that medical school in California that the fat (lipid) in blood could be separated by centrifugation (spinning at high speed).[26-28]

The researchers first removed the red blood cells at low speed and then spun the plasma at ever-higher speeds. The top part, called a fraction, was almost pure fat droplets, which the researchers removed and named chylomicrons. The next four fractions spun at higher speeds were named on their basis of lipid component (fat and cholesterol) as very low density lipoprotein (VLDL), low density lipoprotein (LDL), high density lipoprotein (HDL), and very high density lipoprotein (VHDL). The lipid (fat) content decreased from 90% in the VLDL to 40% in VHDL. The protein content increased from 10% in VLDL to 60% in VHDL. These researchers also found that fat must be combined with protein (apoproteins) in the liver to yield "lipoprotein" to be of use to the body. How these lipoproteins are used in the body is explained in Chapter 2. Because studies had shown that it was the fat in the arteries that was causing heart disease, researchers, and medical professionals concentrated on fat in the diet, ignoring the very important protein connection—fat needs protein to be properly utilized in the body. They had an "easy" way of measuring the fat as cholesterol levels, but not of measuring the protein, since the protein was being used up in the process of "living."

To continue the story, one of the first major studies done on cholesterol levels happened on Tangier Island, an isolated geographic area in Chesapeake Bay whose population had a lot of genetic similarity due to a high rate of inter-marriage.[29] This group had lots of LDL, and genetically did not have the normal level of HDL in their blood. They died young of heart disease! It was named Tangier Disease after the island. That study got researchers excited about the role of cholesterol in heart disease and what LDL and HDL were actually doing. However, for this group, it was the lack of HDL that was the problem, not just the abundance of LDL. The subjects' cholesterol couldn't be removed because they didn't have the HDL to help remove it; their arteries "clogged" up with fat as a result. The HDL should serve as the "completing" mechanism, but this was not present to remove the cholesterol. The end result was that total cholesterol levels in the blood (high LDL levels and low HDL levels) were assumed to be the culprit, when the culprit actually is the lack of the HDL mechanism that provides for the removal of cholesterol. This study in addition to the rabbit study got researchers studying the role of cholesterol in heart disease.

When people see physicians today, their triglyceride levels and total cholesterol scores, LDL levels and HDL levels are often used as health markers.[30] These levels are basically ways of measuring how fat is used in our bodies since it is fat combined with proteins that carry cholesterol. Triglycerides measure the amount of fat in the blood, and a healthy triglyceride level is believed to be below 150 mg/dl. These scores are based on 100 ml of blood.[31] What is missing from these measures is how much protein we have, since neither fat (triglycerides) nor cholesterol can float in the blood unless it is combined with protein. Furthermore, our total level of fat consumption is important, since when we eat fat, ideally it gets used up as a calorie source and not much gets deposited in our bodies.

The American Heart Association (AHA) has set some standards for what are believed to be healthy cholesterol levels. I disagree with those standards! They say

18

that the total cholesterol should be less than 200mg/dl with readings of 200- 239mg/dl, considered moderate risk, and those above 240mg/dl, at higher risk for heart disease. They believe LDL should be less than 100 mg/dl (higher levels would indicate the blood contains too much fat) and HDL greater than 30mg/dl since a lower level indicates not enough HDL is circulating in the body.[31]

LDL is often called "bad" cholesterol and HDL is often called "good" cholesterol, but both labels are incorrect. Labeling cholesterol good or bad should be based on its correct or incorrect use by the body. From my point of view, the right amount of cholesterol is the amount your body needs to maintain itself. This varies from person to person. The public has an overly simplistic view of cholesterol that leads them to believe that simply lowering cholesterol levels reduces heart disease risks. While levels of LDL and HDL are likely to say a great deal about your diet—especially your fat intake—it is your fat intake (both amount and kind) that likely impacts your health in a crucial way. Some physicians believe that a high HDL level helps remove cholesterol from the wall of the artery, although no one is quite certain that it does. It is also not known for sure why more LDL isn't made into HDL—it may be because the body doesn't have enough protein to help make it into an HDL. Or it may be because there is more LDL than any one body can be expected to handle— the capacity has been reached with simply too much fat in the blood. Or it may be another completely different, and as yet unknown, reason or reasons. HDL is a key participant in fat and cholesterol metabolism. However, exactly how HDL works is still a mystery.[32] There is more to the story than LDL, HDL, and triglyceride levels. What I can say is that simply lowering your cholesterol levels does not necessarily lower your risk of heart disease. It is far more complex than that.

How Cholesterol Levels Get Raised (and Lowered)

The daily cholesterol dietary intake of Americans was 600 mg per day from 1909 through 1973. (To put mg or milligrams into context, 10 grains of table salt weigh one milligram.) This amount has dropped to 300-400 mg per day with the AHA recommending a daily allowance of 200 mg/day or lower.[31] I disagree with this recommendation because many cholesterol-containing foods have high nutritional value. Furthermore, even if less dietary cholesterol is consumed, the body still needs cholesterol to stay alive. The liver nevertheless will make enough cholesterol to meet the body's actual daily requirement of approximately 900 mg/day unless its synthesis is inhibited by a statin drug. Statins are a class of drugs used to reduce fat levels in the blood. It is interesting to note that human milk contains very high levels of cholesterol because babies are growing rapidly and need more cholesterol to make cells.[33] If adults consumed as much cholesterol in their food as infants do in human milk per day, they would be ingesting 2650 mg of cholesterol a day, more than the approximately 2000 mg/day an adult actually needs. If cholesterol were not good for us, it would not be in such high concentrations in mother's milk. Cholesterol is good for us!

Experiments conducted on people's diets and cholesterol levels confirm this. Studies focusing on eating eggs showed that eating even three eggs a day did not significantly raise people's cholesterol levels.[34] And when swine were fed rations containing cholesterol, about the equivalent of 40 eggs per day, their blood cholesterol levels did not change significantly.[35] When this diet was modified to include an amount of cholesterol the equivalent of 200 eggs per day, their total blood cholesterols did go up. This suggests that there is an upper limit to how much cholesterol can be ingested.[36] Rats and swine (and people) can easily handle some cholesterol, but not a diet super high in cholesterol. Too much of even the life- sustaining cholesterol is bad!

Other experiments have shown that people's cholesterol levels can be raised by what people eat. Eating saturated fats (animal fats and hydrogenated fats) does raise cholesterol levels. Hydrogenated trans fats raise the cholesterol levels even more than natural trans fats.[37] Eating too many calories from any food sources raises cholesterol levels. Cholesterol levels will also vary depending on how much protein is in the diet.[9] One study varied the amount of fat in the diet while keeping protein amounts the same. The energy/protein ratio (E/P) is a measure of the amount of fat (energy or calories) to the amount of protein; with more fat or calories, the E/P ratio gets worse. With increases in either vegetable or animal fats, this E/P ratio gets worse. The addition of any kind of fat would increase the cholesterol in people already on high fat diets. Some diets have recommended replacing an animal fat with a vegetable fat to decrease cholesterol levels since vegetable fats lower cholesterol levels. However, this is unlikely to solve the problem. The E/P ratio is more important than the kind of fat used in the diet; both kinds of fats can increase cholesterol levels[9] and high amounts of any fat are more of a concern than the type of the fat. (See more on E/P ratios in Chapter 3). Eating animal fats has been equated with elevated cholesterol levels, although this is just one possible way to elevate those levels. In actuality, the U.S. diet has both animal fat and partially hydrogenated vegetable fat which increase the cholesterol level. In summary, cholesterol in the blood can be elevated by these factors:

- Too many total calories in the diet from any source that can be used to make cholesterol, whether the calories come from sugar, starch, protein, or vegetable or animal fat.

- Too many calories from hydrogenated trans fat.
- Not enough or an imbalance of the amino acids (proteins).

Cholesterol and Heart Disease

Thousands of studies have been conducted trying to relate the origin of heart disease to diet, often specifically to cholesterol levels; some looked at what raises cholesterol in the first place and others focused more specifically on cholesterol itself. None have shown that cholesterol causes heart disease. The following paragraphs review some of the studies. Dr. Henry McGill[38] looked for the trends in this "diet-causing heart disease" hypothesis reviewing hundreds of studies from 1950-1979. He found the number of studies increasing dramatically, but no definite answers emerged. One of the problems with many studies was the precision and accuracy of cholesterol determinations in many of the laboratories of that time. In these studies, he noted that diet, specifically high cholesterol levels, did not explain heart disease. Mortality rates due to heart disease continued to rise in technically developed countries. Dr. McGill labeled the decade between 1960-1969 as the "Golden Age" of experimentation on the effects of dietary cholesterol on atherosclerosis and cholesterol concentration. More reports appeared describing an effect of dietary cholesterol on cholesterol concentration, and several studies included larger numbers of subjects and better control of other dietary components, particularly fat.

It was clear from controlled experiments in humans that cholesterol uptake did influence blood cholesterol concentration, and eating saturated fats (animal or hydrogenated fats) increased the cholesterol level even more. However, uncertainty remained regarding how large the effect really was. And there was also uncertainty about the actual effects of ingesting different amounts of

22

cholesterol, the different types of saturated fat, e.g., natural animal fat in contrast with trans (hydrogenated) fat, and the form of the fat. None of the larger studies showed that cholesterol concentrations were appreciably affected by the dietary cholesterol, including saturated fats.

Despite the repeated demonstrations of the mixed and often small effect of dietary cholesterol on blood cholesterol in the previous decade, controversy continued and additional experiments were conducted to explore its effects under various conditions and in various types of subjects. Based on his review of hundreds of studies, Dr. McGill concluded that numerous studies have failed to find a significant independent association of dietary cholesterol with either plasma (blood) cholesterol concentration or with risk of heart disease.

In Great Britain, another researcher also looked at studies on heart disease and diet. Dr. A.S. Truswell[39] stated that plasma cholesterol can be lowered in most people with high or average cholesterol levels by reducing the saturated fat and cholesterol of the diet. Fat in the diet does increase cholesterol levels, but the effect is small with individual variation. The first 300 milligrams of dietary cholesterol have the greatest effect on cholesterol levels. He commented that most of the expert committees considering dietary recommendations had recommended reducing dietary cholesterol to 300 milligrams per day, but that several had not made such a recommendation. He concluded that, at least in Britain, the effect of reducing dietary cholesterol by halving egg intake (from about 4 or 5 to about 2 per person per week) would be so small that this recommendation was not advisable. These studies did demonstrate that cholesterol levels can be altered through diet. However, the direct link between the plasma cholesterol level and heart attacks was not shown in these studies.

The cholesterol hypothesis gained more evidence from epidemiological studies, which made much of the fact that heart disease is more prevalent in affluent, industrial nations where the diet is rich in animal products and comparatively rare in the Far East and in undeveloped countries where animal protein plays a smaller part in the diet. However, there are many other factors in the diet that could account for these differences such as the effects of total calories eaten per day, the effects of ingesting hydrogenated trans fats, differences in certain mineral intakes and life expectancy. The funding of research showing that "cholesterol is bad" became abundant. That statement became well known in part because it was easy to understand and to market. This interpretation became an accepted fact that is still prevalent today. Measuring the cholesterol in our blood and in our food became a standard practice.

The conventional preventive approach developed for lowering the risk of heart disease involved monitoring the amount of saturated fat and cholesterol in the diet. Eating little saturated fat and maintaining low cholesterol levels were recommended.[39] This meant reducing the consumption of meat and meat products, dairy foods, and especially eggs, all of which contain cholesterol. It also meant replacing saturated animal fat, such as butter, with saturated fat made from vegetable oil produced by hydrogenation, such as margarine. This dietary approach was generally familiar to most people both through the medical advice they were given and through television and magazine advertisements for margarines, vegetable oils, and shortenings and a number of vegetable protein meat- and egg-substitutes. Even today, the words "no cholesterol" on the label of a food item helps sell it, even if that food in any form never contained cholesterol in the first place. Much of the research on heart disease has concentrated on diet as the culprit in heart disease, particularly high dietary cholesterol levels; this is the traditional or cholesterol hypothesis. As a consequence, many people try to alter their diets and take drugs to lower

24

the cholesterol levels in their blood. Yet, this has not worked to prevent heart disease.

Concerns About Cholesterol-Lowering Drugs

An additional approach to lowering cholesterol levels is to use drugs that will do this in the body. "Although there is not, and never has been, any convincing evidence that levels of serum (or plasma) cholesterol have any causal relationship with coronary heart disease, that hasn't stopped the cholesterol hypothesis being used as a basis for the sale of drugs to lower blood cholesterol levels."[40] Over the last 65 years, a whole range of drugs has been tried. All, without exception, were unsuccessful in preventing death even while they were successful in lowering cholesterol levels in the blood. No unequivocal evidence was produced that cholesterol lowering, whether by diet or various drugs, extends life or reduces overall mortality. For example, an older drug, cholestyramine inhibits cholesterol absorption from the intestinal tract.[41] In one of its major trials, there was only a difference of 3 deaths; 68 in the group fed cholestyramine and 71 in the placebo group. Cholestyramine never became a popular drug as it was difficult to consume, and its results were not dramatic. These cholesterol-lowering drugs work in a variety of ways; some inhibit the production of cholesterol in the liver and others, the absorption of cholesterol in the intestine. Patents covering these drugs last for 20 years; when a patent is about to expire, often the drug company will come up with a "new" cholesterol-lowering drug so as to maintain its market share.

With any drug, it is important to note its chemical structure as well as its side effects. Here is the most notable example. In the 1950s one cholesterol-lowering drug, triparanol, was in use. It inhibited the synthesis of cholesterol in the liver in the last step in the long number of steps that results in its distribution in the blood plasma. Five years after its introduction, victims of heart disease who had taken the drug began to go blind, and they automatically received compensation from the company that distributed it. These tragic results could have been prevented if the drug's chemical structure had been more carefully scrutinized. Triparanol was closely related in chemical structure to the insecticide DDT that was causing so many problems at the time and has since been banned in the U.S. Both triparanol and DDT contain chlorine in their chemical makeup. The problem was how triparanol worked in the last steps in the synthesis of cholesterol in the liver, when a cholesterol derivative called desmosterol is supposed to be converted to cholesterol, but wasn't. The method used to detect cholesterol at the time couldn't detect desmosterol. The eye contains a high concentration of cholesterol, and desmosterol could not serve as a substitute for cholesterol. Desmosterol caused the lens to become opaque, somewhat similar to macular degeneration in the eye. Desmosterol could serve as a substitute for cholesterol in other bodily functions, but not in the eye.

A number of other drugs on the market are being used to lower blood cholesterol levels. One is Lovastatin, a cholesterol-lowering drug developed from a mold. One researcher found this drug inhibited the use of coenzyme Q,[42] which is a necessary vitamin in converting the energy in foods to energy needed in the body.[43,44] This could have a longer-term detrimental effect on the body. Another researcher found that statin use inhibited the production of prostacyclin, needed to keep the blood flowing.[45] A U.S. firm bought the patent for Lovastatin but since patents are good only for 20 years, they created another statin by changing the chemical structure of Lovastatin slightly. Another US firm has a similar patented statin. Cholesterol-lowering drugs are used worldwide and are a multi-billion-dollar a year industry.[46] Cholesterol-lowering drugs often work by inhibiting the liver in its cholesterol-making role. A concern is that they may do too good of a job and cause the

26

liver to make lower amounts than what the body needs. Remember cholesterol is needed to make cells, including the construction of muscle cells. A common side effect of statins is weak muscles (myopathy),[47] and this occurs because cells may not be able to make muscle tissue without cholesterol. There is no documentation to date on the influence of these drugs on the synthesis of actual muscle cells of the heart that are needed to keep it beating.

One of the issues with the research on the effects of statins is what the subject's heart is like in the first place. Neither high nor low cholesterol levels equate to a healthy heart. Unfortunately I can speak to the latter case personally. I had a low cholesterol level all my life and passed the treadmill test with flying colors when I was close to 90. It was only with an echocardiogram that something showed up wrong, and then the cardiac catheterization indicated blockages. I required coronary by-pass surgery.

Studies of the long-term effect of statins are expensive, and often supported by the drug company with a vested interest in the outcome. From personal experience, I tried to obtain one cholesterol-lowering drug (a statin) from the manufacturer for research purposes. I was asked to sign a three-page document requiring me to submit the results of my research to the company three weeks prior to submitting the research paper to a journal. I could not, in good conscience, conduct research with such restrictions. Another problem with these studies is the length of time of the study; most are based on only a few months to a few years follow-up, not a long enough period of time to evaluate the long-term effects of a drug. For example, one study looked at a statin's effect over a three week period; this is simply not a long enough time period to study this drug's effect.[48]

One study on statins often quoted in research articles is a 1994 one on 4,444 patients in Scandinavian countries.[49] It was designed to evaluate the effect of using a statin to lower cholesterol levels on the mortality of patients with symptoms of heart disease. The study followed 2,221 patients on the statin and 2,223 patients on a placebo (a "fake" drug) for an average of 5.4 years. The data has been analyzed in a number of ways, comparing survivorship rates with deaths from heart attacks and deaths from all causes in both groups and separating the women's data from the men's. This 1994 study[49] is the "flagship" of many studies on statins because it was the only one that focused on definite death from heart attacks for a long enough period of time to provide such data.

On the surface, it looks like statins made a difference. However, looking deeper into the study, some interesting information about the baseline characteristics of the sample in the paper surfaces. The patients were very well randomized on the basis of sex, age and symptoms of heart disease with the result that there were similar numbers in both the statin and placebo groups. However, they were not randomized on the basis of smoking history. It is well established that smoking is a significant risk factor in heart disease.[50,51] There were 54 fewer smokers and 56 more ex-smokers in the statin group than in the placebo group. If the patients had been randomized on the basis of smoking history, there may have been less difference between the placebo and statin groups. Of the 4,444 patients, there were 30 definite deaths from heart attacks in the statin group and 63 in the placebo group. It would have only taken a shift of 17 people with a smoking history from the placebo group to the statin group to potentially provide one more death in the statin group than the placebo group. As no data was provided on the definite observed death from heart attacks between smokers and non-smokers, this well planned study is not as conclusive as it could have been.

Although the study was planned to test only definite observed death from heart attacks between the statin and placebo groups, the statistical analysis was based on total deaths from all causes and showed statistically more deaths in the placebo than the statin group. The data presented on cerebrovascular (stroke) deaths, actually showed two more in the statin than the placebo group or 14 and 12 respectively. Since atherosclerosis causes the same problems in both cerebral and coronary arteries, one would expect statins to significantly lower cerebrovascular deaths as well. They did not. Overall deaths in the women had 25 dying in the placebo group and 27 dying in the statin group, although we do not know specifically how many died of heart disease.

A Swedish study of four million people concluded statins have no effect on atherosclerosis. Other studies show that statins do lower inflammation, a factor some consider important in heart disease.[52] The studies on statins show different results; however, none have proven that statins prevent heart disease.[53-58] Some studies on statins agreed that statins do lower cholesterol levels. However, lower cholesterol levels have not eliminated deaths from heart disease. Existing drugs to aggressively treat cholesterol levels have not met their goals of preventing death. Recent studies involving a statin indicated that two thirds of heart patients taking a statin received no benefit from it.[59,60] These studies did not indicate what benefits the one-third received.

In summary, the story is not a simple one of taking or not taking a statin or any cholesterol-lowering drug, but a much more complicated one of eating properly over the years, exercising, and having the good fortune to be born with a gene pool that is not as susceptible to heart disease. The way fat and cholesterol are used by the body has not received enough consideration in the attempt to lower CHD.[61] As a colleague, Dr. Laurence Pilgeram, once said to me, "The answer to heart disease is a physiological molecule for which basic research is required and not a patentable non-physiologic designer drug." What these cholesterol-lowering drugs are actually doing to the body in the long run, even longer than five years, needs to be well documented. For example, it took longer than five years for the deleterious effects of estrogen on breast cancer to be detected. By focusing on lowering cholesterol levels, we may possibly be creating health problems in the future.

Research on Heart Disease

In conducting research on heart disease, one route is to experimentally create conditions mimicking heart disease in animals and compare their disease with that of humans.[62] Pathologists in my laboratory have found signs of fatty streaks in the arteries even before birth, not only in humans[63-67] but in swine that have a similar circulatory system to humans.[68-78] People (and swine) seem destined to develop at least some atherosclerosis during their lifetime; it even begins in the womb. Dr. Hideshige Imai, one of the world's experts in using an electron microscope, and Dr. Taura could not tell the difference between the coronary arteries of a five- year-old swine (considered "old age" for a swine) on a "regular" diet, free of cholesterol, from that of a 60- year-old man who died of heart disease.[75-81] Thus, aging was a significant risk factor in heart disease in swine as well as man. It was also possible to increase atherosclerosis in swine whenever the normal diet was altered by adding hydrogenated fat or by increasing the amounts of vitamin D[79-84], sugar, or egg yolk powder or by decreasing magnesium in the diet. Arteries from these swine looked just like those of human arteries with heart disease. Thus we "created" heart disease by simply aging or altering the diet.

Another step in heart disease research was to see what actually happens in the arterial cells during the development of that disease. Remember that atherosclerosis first occurred at the branching points of the coronary arteries. We determined the chemical composition of the cells at both the branching and non- branching sections of the arteries. That chemical analysis identified four elements: phospholipids, cholesterol, calcium, and fatty acid content.

We used swine fed a diet that was free of cholesterol and saturated fat.[75] There were two key results. First, age made a difference. The older swine had more build-up of one component, a phospholipid named sphingomyelin, in their arteries. Other studies show that sphingomyelin is important in promoting heart disease because it allows more calcium to incorporate itself into the cell and thus contributes to hardening of the artery.[20] The second result of this study, comparing the phospholipid composition of the branching and non-branching segments of the swine's arteries, found that the cells from the branching segments had even more sphingomyelin than the non-branching cells.[20]

The next step was to look at human cells for evidence of heart disease:

- The branching and non-branching sections of human arteries were compared with the branching segments having more sphingomyelin than the non- branching segments.

- The non-branching coronary arteries from men 21-27 years of age and the arterial tissue from umbilical cords of newborns were compared. The cells from the umbilical cords contained only 10% sphingomyelin while those of the non-branching aorta of the young men contained 40% sphingomyelin.

- The arterial cells from women and men with heart disease were analyzed. Subjects ranged in age from 26-76 years and were undergoing elective coronary bypass surgery. Their artery tissue contained up to 50% sphingomyelin. The arteries from younger coronary by-passed men and women had as high a percentage of sphingomyelin in their arteries as in the artery tissue from older by-passed men and women.[20]

These studies indicate that the cell sphingomyelin composition of the arteries is a significant factor in the development of heart disease. It is interesting to note that the arteries of young men contained only 10% less sphingomyelin than artery tissue from older bypassed patients indicating these young men may have had a considerable amount of atherosclerosis in their arteries. Autopsies of young soldiers killed in the Vietnam and Korean wars indicated the presence of considerable amounts of atherosclerosis in their arteries.[85] Two risk factors were substantiated by these data. One, more sphingomyelin and calcium accumulated at the branching sections of arteries and two, the sphingomyelin content of arteries increases with age in humans as well as in swine.

A lack of magnesium[86-102] may also lead to heart disease. Human arterial cells, as well as the arterial cells and tissue from chicken, swine, and rats that were fed magnesium deficient diets showed more signs of atherosclerosis. A deficiency in vitamin B_6 [103,104] also may contribute to heart disease. Vitamin B_6 is important because it is necessary in the metabolism of amino acids (protein). When vitamin B_6 is missing, cholesterol cannot be properly metabolized. (See Chapter 6 for more on vitamins).

Now that we've gone through some of the experimental research documenting how and where heart disease develops, let's look at some additional facts on heart disease. Did you know that:

• The majority of people at a local hospital who needed coronary by-pass surgery because of heart disease actually had low blood cholesterol levels (below 200 mg).[105]

• Autopsies done in 1936 at a New York hospital on people who had died of sudden death from heart disease showed no correlations with their cholesterol levels.[106]

- Over 65 years of intensive research on cholesterol and heart disease has failed to show that cholesterol causes heart disease.

- Consumption of animal food products, such as milk (which contains cholesterol), was not found to be a clear risk factor. The aortas from Masai in Africa who drink milk as a main source of calories had little atherosclerosis compared to aortas from U.S. citizens who likely consumed more processed foods which probably contained trans fats for their main sources of calories.[107]

An Alternative Explanation of Cholesterol and Heart Disease

Lowering cholesterol levels has not proven to be the answer to preventing heart disease. My research is based on the biochemistry of heart disease. In this hypothesis, the biochemistry of cholesterol serves as a means of explaining heart disease. This will be discussed later with diet recommendations that may make a difference in the development of heart disease in you. The actual way cholesterol is used by the body, not the way cholesterol gets into the body in the first place (through diet or through being made by the liver) will provide that answer. In this scenario, "good" cholesterol is unoxidized cholesterol that comes either from your food or is made by your liver. Good cholesterol is used by the enzymes in the cell to make new cells. "Bad" cholesterol is actually cholesterol that has been oxidized or transformed into a new compound and is misused in the body. Complicating the story is the fact that some of those oxidized cholesterol forms are good, while others are bad!

The question to be answered is how "good" cholesterol turns into "bad" cholesterol,[108-110] and we're not talking about LDL and HDL here. Cholesterol actually takes on two different forms based on how it is used (or oxidized) in the body. One form is the unoxidized cholesterol because its molecular structure contains no added oxygen. This unoxidized cholesterol is present both in animal products such as eggs, meat, and dairy products and in every cell membrane of the 50,000 trillion cells that compose our body. It is also present in the cells of animals and sea life, such as chickens, cows, swine, sheep, fish, shrimp, and lobsters, all of which are sources of food that contain cholesterol. This form of cholesterol is clearly life-giving, and it's truly the "good" cholesterol. Cholesterol's second form (an oxysterol) is the cholesterol in the blood (and tissue) that has taken on extra oxygen in its molecular structure. Many oxysterols, produced in the liver, are necessary for the process of "life" in our bodies, but some are not.[111-116] When cholesterol is oxidized, at least 40 different derivatives, or kinds of oxysterols, are created.[117]

Structural integrities of these oxidized cholesterols are relatively unstable; however, these molecules have multiple purposes, some good, and some not so good. These oxidized cholesterols can function as important precursors for some of the most essential steroid hormones in the body, including for example, testosterone, estrogen, progesterone, and cortisol. Cholesterol converted to bile acids helps in the absorption of fat from the intestinal tract. Still other kinds of oxysterols serve to regulate the amount of unoxidized cholesterol in the LDL made by our liver. However, at least seven "lethal" oxysterols are present in excess amounts in the blood of patients with coronary heart disease.[118-121] Two of these "bad" oxysterols come from the diet and can easily be avoided, such as those produced in fried foods and powdered egg yolks.[121] The other five lethal oxysterols are due to the dysfunctional metabolism of cholesterol in the liver when excess oxysterols are present; thus these can be avoided by eating a proper diet. This approach to cholesterol and heart disease then focuses on the biochemistry involved and looks at the actual chemical composition of the diseased cells and what causes that change from healthy to unhealthy cells.[62,64] As you can see, this section has scientific aspects to it, but please bear with the science since it does explain a lot of what happens with cholesterol.

The cholesterol hypothesis suggests that high cholesterol levels are responsible for the formation of atherosclerosis.[30] Studying the effects of high cholesterol levels on the severity of atherosclerosis is one way to check this hypothesis.[122] The previous research seemed to suggest that the high cholesterol level (high LDL) was responsible for causing atherosclerosis. We used a specific kind of chicken for the study, one with a genetic defect that led to extremely high blood cholesterol levels and the development of heart disease within two years.[119-127] We fed half the chickens vitamin E (an antioxidant). Sure enough, these chickens still had high cholesterol levels but they had less atherosclerosis in their arteries because of the vitamin E than the chickens that did not get the vitamin E. This indicates that it was a high oxidation level, not the high cholesterol level, that was responsible for the atherosclerosis.[122]

To trigger the conditions that lead to atherosclerosis, research studies[128,129] indicate that low density lipoprotein (LDL) must be modified to oxidized LDL (oxLDL). Thus oxysterols as a component of oxLDL is truly the bad cholesterol; LDL, per se, is a natural, good part of our blood. The increase in oxLDL correlated not only with the extent of coronary blockage, but also with the development of that blockage called stenosis. These oxidation products induced damage of cellular membrane[111,112] and produced an increase in plaques and calcium.[115,130] An increase in calcium was found in the arteries, especially at the branches, and led to irreversible changes in the arteries.

The body tries to meet this oxidative challenge with a host of defense mechanisms including vitamins (particularly C, E, and B_6), enzymes and albumin. Albumin functions as a carrier of bile pigments, the by-products of cholesterol metabolism. One of these bile pigments is called bilirubin.[131-133] Another protein in the blood named fibrinogens is also an efficient antioxidant[134] preventing superoxides, and other "bad" by-products, from forming. Fibrinogens, albumin, and two other proteins in the blood named ceruloplasmin and transferrin act as a supplementary defense mechanism against oxidative stress. This oxidative stress leads to inflammatory conditions, similar to how a fever indicates an infection in the body. These inflammatory conditions are now believed to be a symptom of heart disease.

Oxysterols are potent oxidizing agents that can alter the lipid composition of blood vessels and lead to heart disease.[105] In a study on 2,000 patients diagnosed with heart disease, cholesterol levels ranged from 100-380. Of those requiring by-pass surgery because of blockages of 75% or higher, only 15% of the men and 33% of the women had cholesterol levels over 240, considered the high-risk category. Cholesterol levels thus did not correlate with the extent of stenosis (blockage) in the coronary arteries of these patients. However, all 2,000 patients had higher concentrations of lipid oxidation products, higher concentrations of acute phase proteins (a sign of heart disease) and lower total antioxidant capacity in their blood than age and sex matched patients without apparent blockage of their coronary arteries. All of the cardiac patients had higher concentrations of an amino acid, homocysteine, in their blood than age and sex matched controls. The higher homocysteine levels may be due to a deficiency of vitamin B_6 in our diets. Since oxysterols formed by oxidation of cholesterol were detected as oxidation products in oxLDL, we hypothesized that the oxysterols in oxLDL were responsible for arterial cell injury and for the development of atherosclerosis and calcification at the cellular level in patients with severe heart disease.

We showed earlier that cell membranes change during a lifetime.[20] It is a natural process for all of us to develop at least some hardening of the arteries. One way to show this change more dramatically is to study the veins of coronary artery by-passed patients.[135] By-pass procedures include finding veins in legs or perhaps arteries in arms that can be harvested or cut out and then use those to by-pass the diseased arteries leading to the heart. Of particular interest is the chemical composition of the veins that have been used as arteries to the heart in people who require a second by-pass operation. These veins in the first by-pass surgery were obviously clear when they were used to substitute for the arteries into the heart. They contained 10% sphingomyelin and 50% phosphatidylcholine.

However, in this group of second time by-pass patients, those veins also became "clogged" and needed replacement. The vein that substituted for the clogged artery got clogged itself and the "debris" (calcified deposit) was as bad as that in the original bad artery. By studying the chemical composition of those veins, we found that changes occurred in these veins acting like arteries causing calcium deposits in them. The cell membrane composition of the clogged vein indicated it contained 40 times more calcium as well as significantly more sphingomyelin than the native vein. The replacement vein used in the second by-pass was not clogged and its cell membrane composition was normal. The failed vein contained 50% sphingomyelin and 20% phosphatidylcholine.

To further check this result of cells becoming calcified, we grew human cells along with a "lethal" oxysterol.[20] Those cells cultured with a "lethal" oxysterol changed and resembled the composition of the clogged vein of the second bypass surgery. That we could repeat in the laboratory the same biochemical changes that were found in the veins of bypassed patients showed that oxysterols are a risk factor in heart disease. The changes in the cell structure allowed calcium to flow into the arterial cell and disrupted its normal functioning. Calcium remains embedded in the cell walls of the arteries. It is that calcium and sphingomyelin that eventually leads to coronary heart disease. In humans, excess oxysterols stimulated the synthesis of sphingomyelin.

By using a radioactive choline, the time- and dose-dependent effects of oxysterols on sphingomyelin synthesis could be observed. Oxysterols at a level of 0.1µg/mL, a very small amount, which is within the range of its plasma concentration in healthy adults, had no obviously stimulating effect on the incorporation of choline label into sphingomyelin from phosphatidylcholine (one of the five components of the cellular membrane) during 15 days of treatment. When the level was increased to 0·5µg/mL, however, it took only 3 days for oxysterols to stimulate an increase in radioactivity in sphingomyelin indicating that the sphingomyelin came from phosphatidylcholine.[136,137]

These results indicate that oxysterols increase the transfer of choline from phosphatidylcholine into sphingomyelin when it is present in concentrations higher than those found in healthy adults. This was consistent with the reports that both oxysterols and sphingomyelin increase in atherosclerosis.[138]

Therefore, this explains why oxysterols, sphingomyelin and calcium levels are high in the coronary arteries of bypass surgery patients.

In summary, my hypothesis for the cause of heart disease and sudden coronary death is based on the composition, structure, and biochemistry of the coronary arteries and veins. The main generator of atherosclerosis and sudden death are oxysterols in excess. As shown in my laboratory, normal levels of oxysterols in the plasma will not cause phosphatidylcholine to convert into sphingomyelin and therefore less calcium will bind to the arterial wall, resulting in fewer blockages in the arteries, which will reduce the occurrence and risk of sudden cardiac death.

CHAPTER 1: Key Points

- Cholesterol is life-sustaining, even though it is not a nutrient. It is essential for the making of the 50,000 trillion cells in the body.
- Cholesterol is either made in the body by the liver or comes as part of food, and it is needed daily.
- People seem to vary in how much cholesterol they naturally have in their systems. There is no one right amount for everyone.
- Cholesterol from our food is seen in the public eye as causing heart disease, yet over 65 years of studies have not proven this to be the case. People with heart disease have varying cholesterol levels.
- Efforts to lower cholesterol may be causing more harm than good.
- By reducing foods high in cholesterol, good nutrition is harder to achieve.
- By taking drugs to lower cholesterol, the capacity to make new cells needed by our bodies is diminished.
- The culprit in heart disease is an excess amount of oxidized cholesterol.
- To help use cholesterol in the body properly, a diet with the proper amounts of protein and fat, low in vitamin D, void of trans fat, and with proper amounts of vitamin B and magnesium is needed.

CHAPTER 2: Eating Fat is Good for You! (Provided it is Not a "Manufactured" Trans Fat)

Fat is probably the most maligned food group in our diet. When people think about eating fat, they usually think about gaining weight and getting fat. However, did you know that:

- Fat is an essential part of any diet—without fat, people cannot live.
- Two types of fats are healthy for you—saturated fat from animals and unsaturated fats from vegetables sources.
- Your body needs both saturated and unsaturated fats to function well.
- There are two types of trans fats—trans fat from the saturated fat of animals and trans fats produced artificially by hydrogenation from vegetable oil. They are used differently in the body with only the latter producing some unhealthy effects.
- Frying food in fat can be done in a healthy way, but current practices are often unhealthy.

Fat contains more than simply fat and cholesterol. It has some key roles in nutrition in the body. These include:

- Providing two essential fatty acids called linoleic (omega-6 or n-6) and linolenic (omega-3 or n-3) acids that are required in human body functioning including reproduction, cell structure, brain function, vision, and blood fluidity and clotting.
- Supplying energy.
- Aiding absorption of vitamins A, D, E, and K, and carotenoids.

41

- Holding your organs, including your kidneys, in place.

Because fat is the main source of unwanted calories in the American diet, its value has been overlooked. First, here is some background on the sources of fat and the fat industry.

Sources of Fat

Fat is supplied to the American diet by three different industries: the animal food industry, the vegetable food industry, and the hydrogenated fat industry.[139-141] The animal food industry supplies the invisible fat as a component of milk, cheese, eggs, and meat as well as visible animal fat such as butter, lard, and tallow. The vegetable fat industry supplies the fat for the production of foods such as salad oils. The hydrogenated fat industry converts vegetable oil to a solid fat by means of hydrogenation: trans fat is made when hydrogen is added to vegetable cooking oil, which increases the shelf life and flavor of foods containing these oils. This industry converts vegetable oil to a hard fat similar to animal fat to produce shortening, margarine, and commercial frying fats.

The fat in corn, canola, cottonseed, or soybeans is a soft fat or a liquid at room temperature and is called unsaturated. There are two types of unsaturated fats based on their chemical structure—monounsaturated fats from a source such as olive oil and polyunsaturated fats from sources like corn oil or soybean oil. The fat in meat or milk is considered a saturated or hard fat since it is a solid at room temperature. The chemistry of the difference between saturated and unsaturated fats has to do with the fact that hard fats melt at a higher temperature (somewhat higher than even body temperature) than do soft fats. Hard and soft fats are both triglycerides because they have three fatty acids attached to one glycerol molecule. Both hard and soft fats have the same caloric (or heat and energy producing) value.

Table 1 shows the consumption of both saturated and unsaturated fats over the last 100 years in the U.S. We have increased the consumption of polyunsaturated fats from 11.3 lb. per capita in 1912 to 64.5 lb per capita in 2011. On the other hand we have decreased the consumption of saturated fats from 28 lb. per capita in 1912 to 13.4 lb. per capita in 2011. This shift, both the increase in total fat consumption and the shift from more saturated fats to unsaturated ones, has had negative consequences for our health. We likely have gained unnecessary weight and created more difficulties in keeping our blood flowing.

Table 1. Fats and vegetable oils consumption in US since 1912 per capita (in pounds)

Years	1912		1950		1999		2011	
Items	Total*	Per cap	Total*	Per cap	Total*	Per cap.	Total*	Per cap
Corn oil	53.0	0.6	223.0	1.47	1416.9	5.2	1620.0	5.2
Cottonseed oil	950.0	10.0	1445.0	9.51	832.8	3.1	620.0	2.0
Olive oil	43.0	0.5	76.0	0.50	329.8	1.2	650.1	2.1
Palm oil	0.0	0.0	26.0	0.17	416	1.5	2525.2	8.1
Palm kernel oil	0.0	0.0	26.0	0.17	233.2	0.9	778.0	2.5
Peanut oil	8.0	0.1	103.0	0.68	1524.7	5.6	202.7	0.6
Canola oil	0.0	0.0	0.0	0.00	111.2	0.4	4249.0	13.6
Safflower oil	0.0	0.0	5.1	0.03	15.8	0.1	60.9	0.2
Sesame oil	0.0	0.0	5.0	0.03	15.8	0.1	27.2	0.1
Soybean oil	16.0	0.2	1446.0	9.51	8029.6	29.4	9000.0	28.8
Sunflower oil	0.0	0.0	0.5	0.00	393.7	1.4	395	1.3
Total unsaturated oils	1070.0	11.3	3355.6	22.1	13319.5	48.8	20128.1	64.5
Lard	1069.0	11.2	1891.0	12.60	202.0	0.7	480.0	1.5
Butter	1579.0	16.6	1648.0	10.70	1307.0	4.8	1510.0	4.8
Tallow	22.0	0.2	69.0	0.45	996.0	3.6	1050.0	3.4
Coconut	0.0	0.0	69.0	0.45	927.0	3.4	1155.1	3.7
Total saturated fats	2670.0	28.0	3677.0	24.2	3432.0	12.6	4195.1	13.4
US Population in millions	95		152		273		312	

(*) Totals in millions of pounds
Courtesy Mark Ash, of U.S. Department of Agriculture, Washington, D.C.
http://factfinder2.census.gov/faces/tableservices/jsf/pages/productview.xhtml?pid=ACS_11_1YR_DP05&prodType=table.
http://www.npg.org/facts/us_historical_pops.htm.
http://www.census.gov/population/estimates/state/st-99-1.txt

Essential Fatty Acids

Fats in the diet provide linoleic and linolenic acid, the "essential" fatty acids for life. These two fatty acids, like the essential amino acids cannot be made in the human body from protein, carbohydrates or other fatty acids. They must be provided in our food. These also have more common names based on their chemical structures. Linolenic acid is also referred to as n-3 or omega-3. Linoleic acid is also called n-6 or omega-6. The amount of these fatty acids needed daily varies by age. Table 2 shows the amounts needed at various ages although I am concerned that these levels may be too high. You don't need much of these essential fatty acids, but you do need some.

Table 2. Daily Recommended Allowances of the Essential Fatty Acids[142]

Gender, Age	Omega-3/n-3 (grams*)	Omega-6/n-6 (grams*)
Children, ages 4-8	0.9 grams	10 grams
Teenagers		
Boys, 14-18	1.6	16
Girls, 14-18	1.1	11
Adults		
Men, 19-50	1.6	17
Men, over 50	1.6	14
Women, 19-50	1.1	12
Women, over 50	1.1	11

*As a point of reference, 28.5 grams = 1 ounce. Four ounces is the equivalent of one stick of butter or 1/2 cup, or 8 tablespoons, or 125 grams.

This data was obtained from the Institute of Medicine National Academy of Science's Dietary Reference Intake Part 1 from 2003.

Once you are convinced that you do need to consume some fats, the next question is what food sources provide them. Table 3 contains some food sources. You'll note that vegetable oils are on the table, but I do not recommend them as sources. This is because they have been heated

45

excessively in their processing, thus stripping them of valuable nutrients. It is best to get your essential fats from food sources other than oils.

Table 3. The Essential Fatty Acids in Various Food Sources[142]

Food (serving size)	Linoleic Acid Omega-3/n-3 (g)	Linoleic Acid Omega-6/n-6 (g)
Oils		
Canola Oil, 1 Tbsp	1.6	3.2
Walnut Oil, 1 Tbsp	1.4	7.6
Soybean Oil, 1 Tbsp	1.0	7.0
Corn Oil, 1 Tbsp	0.9	5.7
Olive Oil, 1 Tbsp	0.6	1.0
Coconut Oil, 1 Tbsp	0.0	0.0
Nuts and Seeds		
Walnut (English), 2 Tbsp	1.0	5.4
Macadamia, 2 Tbsp	1.0	0.0
Vegetables, Fruits, and Legumes		
Soybeans, Cooked, 1 cup	1.1	7.8
Tofu, firm, 1/2 cup	0.7	5.0
Tofu, medium, 1/2 cup	0.4	2.9
Soy milk, 1 cup	0.4	2.9
Berries, 1 cup	0.2	0.2
Peas, 1/2 cup	0.2	0.2
Legumes, 1/2 cup	0.05	0.05
Grains		
Oat germ, 2 Tbsp	0.2	1.6
Wheat germ, 2 Tbsp	0.1	0.8
Meats		
Beef, 100 g	0.3	0.29
Lamb, 100 g	0.06	0.51
Chicken, 100 g	0.03	0.66
Pork, 100 g	0.38	1.12
Fish (Mackerel), 100 g	0.04	0.04
Butter, 1 Tbsp	1.16	2.11

The Role of Essential Fatty Acids

The essential fatty acids serve as sources, or rather precursors, for blood fluidity regulators. The scientific explanation follows. Linoleic acid (n-6) is made (synthesized in the body) into arachidonic acid and then prostacyclin or thromboxane.[143] Prostacyclin and thromboxane have to be continually made from the essential fatty acids because they last only about 10 seconds in the blood and thus must be constantly replaced. Prostacyclin is synthesized in endothelial cells in the blood vessel wall. Thromboxane is synthesized in the platelets in the blood. Your body cannot store prostacyclin or thromboxane, but you can store the essential fatty acids from which they are made. One of those regulators, prostacyclin, keeps the blood fluid, and the other, thromboxane, clots the blood, and there is a complex balance between the two. Blood needs to flow smoothly all the time and to clot only when there is a cut in the skin or if there is an aneurysm, a break in the artery itself. As you can see from Figure 1, this is a complicated process.

Figure 1: Synthesis of Prostacyclin and Thromboxane

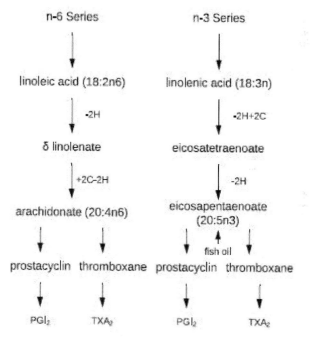

Linolenic acid (n-3) is made into eicosapentaenoic acid for clotting. That in turn is made into prostacyclin and thromboxane. Fish have already converted the linolenic acid they get from seaweed into eicosapentaenoic acid; Figure 1

shows that several steps can be skipped if fish oil is consumed. Hence fish oil is often recommended as a dietary supplement, although as the figure 1 also shows, prostacyclin can come from linolenic acid as well.

The balance between the prostacyclin for flow and thromboxane for clotting is a very delicate one and can be changed by different diets and different drug prescriptions. For example, Coumadin (Warfarin) may be prescribed for those who have heart disease to keep their blood from clotting. However, Coumadin plus the natural production of prostacyclin may cause too much bleeding.[144] This can lead to macular degeneration, an eye disease in which the optic nerve is affected, or excessive nose bleeding or internal bleeding. Vitamin K may be recommended when the blood is too fluid, although it often is in the diet, especially in greens. Vitamin K in excess has the opposite effect, creating too much clotting that could lead to heart attacks caused by coronary artery blockages or strokes caused by cerebral (brain) artery blockages.[145] Vioxx, a medication to alleviate the pain of arthritis, was withdrawn from the market because of its effect on diseases such as heart attacks and strokes; it led to too little production of prostacyclin for fluidity and too much production of thromboxane for clotting.[146]

Essential fatty acids do more than regulate the blood; they are also a key to reproduction. Since the 1930s, we've known that reproduction always fails on fat-free diets.[147] In studies on rats, reproduction continues under low fat conditions because the rats have enough linoleic acid stored in their bodies.[148] They manufacture arachidonic acid from the linoleic acid in their own fat, so they can reproduce healthy young, even after a fat-free diet. If the rats did not have enough linoleic acid stored in their bodies (such as rats born to mothers on fat-free diets), we found they could not make enough of the arachidonic acid needed for healthy reproduction, and their young die. Women need the essential fatty acids for reproduction. The easiest way to supply them is not from the oils but from the other foods listed in table 3.

People also need essential fatty acids for other body functions, such as brain activity and eyesight.[149]Brain cells contain 70% fat including 24% omega-3 and 28% omega-6 fatty acids.[150] Since the body cannot manufacture these, you have to eat the sources of these fats. Fat really is brain food! Calling someone a "fathead" should actually be a compliment! Similarly, the cells of the eye have a high composition of omega-3 and omega-6 fatty acids.[151] It is believed that fatty acids help in the development of vision. Veins and arteries also contain these fatty acids with the veins of adults made up of 5% omega-3 and 6% omega-6 fatty acids.

How Fat is Used in the Body[152]

How fat is used in modern humans was developed in prehistoric humans to assure their survival. There must have been long periods of time between meals, that is, fasting periods, and there were times in which they had food available, the "fed" period. During this fed period, carbohydrates were used within two hours as a quick source of energy. Extra carbohydrates were stored first as glycogen in the muscles and liver and then any excess converted to fat and stored in the adipose tissue (the fat around your middle and elsewhere). This stored fat was then available for energy during the long fasting periods. Modern humans have inherited this way of handling these fed and fasting periods. This process assured the survival of prehistoric humans but has now become one way that obesity is developing in humans today. Too much food is available all hours of the day and night, and eating it is a pleasure.

To avoid adding fat to your body, any carbohydrates you eat should be used up as a calorie source before the next meal. Any carbohydrates that have already turned into fat and any fat in your diet itself should be used for energy within the cell during the fasting period. Eating a snack between meals means adding additional carbohydrates into the system before any of the fat from the previous meal has been used for energy. It ends up adding to your adipose tissue. If you weigh yourself before a hearty meal and again the next day, you may find you have gained a pound or two, the amount depending on how much food you ate and the fat you stored. As such a meal may also contain excess salt, some of the weight gain can be due to excess water you stored. Millions of dollars are spent to try to get rid of this stored fat, and the government is planning to spend millions more dollars to solve the obesity problem. Prehistoric humans had no choice in controlling the time between fasting and fed periods because they had no refrigerators, fast food outlets, or supermarkets to run to. Modern humans do have this choice. More time between the fed periods, that is between meals, may help with the obesity problem.

The fat in the intestinal tract is first converted into tiny droplets of fat (chylomicrons) by the intestinal cells. The intestinal tract is not just a through highway for fat, but is actively involved in the process of metabolizing fat so that the body can use it. The chylomicrons diffuse from the intestinal tract into the lymph system and into the veins through the thoracic duct and end up in the blood. The blood, during the fed period, carries these chylomicrons for deposit where they are resynthesized into adipose tissue and stored fat around the stomach, hips, and other locations. The fat (triglycerides) in adipose tissue is "mobilized" when the glycogen in the muscle and liver has been reduced. These triglycerides get split into glycerin (glycerol) and free fatty acids by an enzyme named hormone sensitive lipase, available for only that purpose.

The glycerin portion goes to the liver. The free fatty acids take a different route and are combined with a protein named albumin. Therefore there must be enough albumin in the blood to "carry" the free fatty acids in the blood.[153,154]

This fatty acid albumin complex is water-soluble enough in the blood to be carried to cells of all kinds that use the fatty acid portion as an energy source. Any excess fatty acid goes to the liver and is remade into triglycerides. The cellular organelle (the endoplasmic reticulum) in the liver cells participates in coating the very small triglyceride droplets with protein and adds phospholipid and cholesterol to produce very low density lipoprotein (VLDL).

VLDL is a main carrier of fat during the fed and fasting periods. Once added to the blood, VLDL gradually loses its triglycerides upon hydrolysis by lipoprotein lipase and eventually winds up as LDL. LDL receptors on tissue cells recognize the LDL, leading to the uptake and utilization of cholesterol in LDL by the cell, according to "the LDL receptor pathway" formulated by Goldstein and Brown for which they received the Nobel Prize in 1985.[155] The triglyceride poor VLDL remnants as well as LDL are enriched with cholesterol ester (a cholesterol plus a fatty acid) transferred from HDL. In the liver, most of the cholesterol is oxidized to cholic acid and eliminated through the intestine. As you can see, the chemical processes of making fat usable are both elegant in their simplicity and complex in their results.

Figure 2. Lipoproteins and Lipids Derived From Fat

Organ	Product
Intestine	Fat in food ↓ Chylomicron
Lymph (blood filtrate)	Chylomicron
Blood	Chylomicron Triglyceride ↓ Depot Triglyceride (Adipose tissue) ↓ Fatty Acid/Albumin Complex VLDL ↓ LDL Cholesterol Ester in HDL ↓ VLDL, LDL
Liver	Apoproteins
	Cholesterol Cholesterol Esters Triglycerides Phospholipids ↓ VLDL LDL Cholesterol ↓ Bile Acids
Intestine	Bile Acids

Hydrogenated Fats and Trans Fats

We've mentioned the three sources of fats—animal fat, vegetable fat, and hydrogenated fat. We've seen how animal and vegetable fats are important to supplying the essential fatty acids. Now it's time to look at the third kind of fat—hydrogenated fats. These are manufactured from unsaturated fats like soybean oil through the process of hydrogenation. This turns a liquid fat into a solid one that stays "fresh" for a longer period of time. This fat serves only as a source of calories or energy our bodies might need and provides no other nutritional value.

First, some history:[156] Before 1910, we had primarily butterfat, beef tallow, and lard in our diets. During Napoleon's reign in France in the early 1800s, a type of margarine was invented to feed the troops using tallow and buttermilk; it did not gain acceptance in the U.S. In the early 1900s, soybeans began to be imported into the U.S. as a source of protein; soybean oil was a by-product. What to do with that oil became an issue. At the same time, there was not enough butterfat available for consumers. The method of hydrogenating fat and turning a liquid fat into a solid one had been discovered, and now the ingredients (soybeans) and the "need" (shortage of butter) were there. Later, the means for storage, the refrigerator, was a factor in trans fat development. The fat industry found that hydrogenated fats provided some special features to margarines, which unlike butter, allowed margarine to be taken out of the refrigerator and immediately spread on a slice of bread. By some minor changes to the chemical composition of hydrogenated fat, they also found such hydrogenated fat provided superior baking properties compared to lard. Margarine made from hydrogenated soybean oil began to replace butterfat. Hydrogenated fat such as Crisco and Spry, sold in England, began to replace lard in the baking of bread, pies, cookies, and cakes in 1920.

Here's the scientific explanation of trans fat with the help of the Food and Drug Administration (FDA). The FDA defines trans fatty acids chemically as "all unsaturated fatty acids that contain one or more isolated (i.e., unconjugated) double bonds in a trans configuration". Unhydrogenated vegetable oils have fatty acids of 18 carbon bonds as in linoleic acid, also known as n-6 or omega-6 and linolenic acid also known as n-3 or omega-3.[157] These two essential fatty acids (EFA) in vegetable oils are unsaturated, that is they have double bonds at 9,12,or 9,12,15 positions on the chain. The hydrogenation process changes the chemical structure of EFA. It causes the migration of the double bonds from 9,12 or 9,12,15 positions to other carbon atoms in the chain producing five positional "cis" isomers or leading to changes of their configuration to become fourteen different trans fatty acids that are not present in animal or vegetable fats. They can serve as a source of energy but they cannot serve as an essential fatty acid.[158] Complete hydrogenation results in stearic acid (a completely saturated fatty acid) and also eliminates the EFA that are necessary in the diet.[159]

The structure of a natural unsaturated fat is called a cis fat. The structure of some cis fat, after hydrogenation, changes into a trans fat. This process also happens in milk-producing animals. For example, grass naturally contains n-3 and n-6 fatty acids. When cows eat the grass, the enzymes in their stomachs change the cis to a trans fat; their butter thus contains 2-4% trans fat. However, this natural trans fat has a different chemical composition than the trans fat produced by industrial hydrogenation. It was assumed by the FDA that the hydrogenation of soybean oil produced the same trans fat chemically and worked the same way in our bodies as the natural trans fat in butter. That is not the case. It took 60 years before the chemical composition was shown to be different[160] and nearly another 10 years before its effects on the body were demonstrated to be different as well.[161]

The exact compositions of the trans fats in partially hydrogenated soybean oil in 1910 were essentially unknown. It was only with the development in 1952 of gas chromatography that the fat composition of hydrogenated fat could be more accurately determined.[162] The necessity of the linoleic (n-6) and linolenic (n-3) fatty acids as essential in the diet had been established by Burr and Burr[147] in 1930; these are the essential fatty acids also called omega-3 and omega-6. Gas chromatography showed that these fatty acids were at low levels in the early hydrogenated fats and that they contained 14 fatty acids that were not present in either animal fats or vegetable oils. For five decades in the U.S., these manufactured fats contained up to 50% trans fat and 11% linoleic acid.[163]

Negative Effects of Manufactured Trans Fats

Dietary studies on coronary heart disease during the 1950s and 1960s looked at trans fats, but for the most part didn't go far enough in studying varying percentages of trans in the hydrogenated fats. Trans fats were metabolized more slowly than natural fats, but whether that was a factor in heart attacks was not shown.[164,165] The National Diet Heart Study, one of the most comprehensive studies on the possible role of dietary fat in heart disease, was carried out in the 1960s.[166] What's important about this study, in hindsight, is that the key to lowering blood cholesterol levels was to decrease the amount of trans in the diet and to increase the amount of linoleic acid, one of the essential fatty acids every human needs to keep blood flowing.[143] Many researchers concluded that consuming margarine was best, not knowing that the essential feature was the increase of linoleic acid in the margarine. The composition of the margarine was the key.

At a conference in 1979, chemists specializing in fats and oils expressed concern about trans fats in the diet[167]; in essence this was a warning to the industry to examine trans fats, but one they did not heed to any great degree. Consumers kept eating trans fats.[168] This dangerous diet continued.

To demonstrate the effect of consuming trans fats, we looked at the composition of pig's heart arteries fed different diets. We fed a group of pregnant swine partially hydrogenated fat that contained 43% trans fat. We also fed two other groups of pregnant swine either corn oil or butter fat. The piglets born to the swine that were fed partially hydrogenated fat contained almost 3% trans fat in their arteries at 8 weeks of age. They contained less arachidonic acid then the piglets born to the other two groups. This indicated their mothers converted less arachidonic acid from linoleic acid. Arachidonic acid is essential to the synthesis of prostacyclin, that keeps the blood flowing. The milk from the swine fed partially hydrogenated fat contained significant amounts of trans fat, which the piglets received when nursing. Piglets born to swine who were fed corn oil or butterfat in their diets had no changes in their arterial developing cells and contained no trans fat .[160]

There is a parallel between the effects of trans fat on pigs and on humans. For example, if a mother is breast-feeding her child and also eating any kind of food with trans fats, she would have a substantial amount of trans fats in her milk supply and pass those to her infant which cause a decrease of arachidonic acid in their arteries.[168] In cases where children died and had been autopsied, 99% showed the beginning stages of hardening (calcifications) of the arteries, which ultimately leads to heart disease.[169,170]

On January 1, 2006, the Food and Drug Administration (FDA) began to require the labeling of foods that contain trans fatty acids.[171] The FDA based this directive on 160 scientific articles that showed bad effects of trans fat. At that time, the FDA did not go far enough. First, it allowed products that have less than 0.5 gram of total trans fat per serving to be exempt as long as no claims are made about fat, fatty acids, or cholesterol content. This is a problem because many people eat more than one serving at a time, and because the effect of even small amounts of trans fat consumption can add up. We collected 15 samples of food items that claimed 0 grams of trans fat. We found one contained 0 grams trans fat, one contained more than .5 grams, and 13 contained just a shade under .5 grams of trans fat. Second, it treated hydrogenated trans fat the same as natural trans fat when in fact they work differently in the body. Trans fats that come from hydrogenated fat change the composition of the arteries while natural trans fats do not.

Trans fats reduce the amount of prostacyclin released by endothelial cells that line the arteries.[136]

On November 7, 2013, the FDA announced that it would ban all manufactured trans fats. Finally my goal has been reached, one that began with my first publication on trans fat in 1957. [21]

Which "table fat" to eat, butter or margarine, has been a source of confusion for the consumer for over 50 years although I have always been clear on this. Butter is a byproduct of the dairy industry and has been consumed for centuries; it is a good source of the needed essential fatty acids. Margarine is a manufactured product created from hydrogenated soybean oil or fish oils. Margarine can be processed so that it does not contain trans fat. However, if we think that all we have to do is eat trans fat free margarines, we still have not solved the problem. Many diets, including those of the American Heart Association and the United States Department of Agriculture (USDA) have recommended margarine rather than butter as the preferred table fat since 1961, advice I have disagreed with ever since. This advice[21] ignores the fact that the human body contains (and needs) both saturated and unsaturated fat, and evidence indicates that unsaturated fat (the essential fatty acids) "cancels out" the influence of saturated fat on blood cholesterol levels. Furthermore, it ignores the fact that hydrogenated trans fats are unhealthy. Butter is actually a healthier product to consume than margarine.

To summarize, the consumption of hydrogenated fats, which are in foods like margarine, and partially hydrogenated soybean oil, can throw off the balance between prostacyclin (needed for blood flow) and thromboxane (needed for clotting) production in the body. Up to this point, the assumption was that adding enough linoleic acid would compensate for what trans fats might be doing to the production of prostacyclin. However, that is not enough to overcome the negative effects of trans fats.

Heart Disease Rates and Trans Fat Consumption

Heart disease death rates were 341 per hundred thousand in 1911. This number increased in every decade and by 1950 it had reached nearly 600 per 100,000. The sharpest declines in heart disease death rates started in 1968. It began decreasing somewhat and by 1970 was 492 per 100,000.[174] So what happened to the death rates from 1910 - 2011? In 1910 oil was partially hydrogenated to produce a fat that was used to replace butterfat and lard and the U.S. population starting eating those fats. The composition of those fats were unknown until the 1950s when gas chromatography could show that those fats contained 14 fatty acids that were not present in either animal fats or vegetable oils.

My concerns on the negative effects of trans fats started in the 1950s, and I began discussing my concerns as a member of the American Heart Association's (AHA) committee on nutrition guidelines. My research was showing that linoleic acid was needed to keep blood flowing and that process was inhibited by the trans fats. I suggested to the Medical Director of the AHA, Dr. Campbell Moses,[175] that he persuade the Institute of Shortening and Edible Oils to change industry standards to lower the trans fat and increase the essential fatty acid composition of margarine and shortening. I have been able to document that this change occurred in 1968.[176] Prior to 1968 margarine contained 43.9% trans acid and 8.4% linoleic acid (an essential fatty acid) while shortening contained 30% trans acid and 8% linoleic acid. After 1968, the industry agreed to lower the trans acids in margarines to 27.7% and shortening to 20%. They also increased the linoleic acid in margarine to 27.3% and shortening to 24%. The heart disease death rates decreased steadily since 1968 to 173.7 per 100,000 in 2011. I believe some of that decrease is due to this changed formulation of the hydrogenated fats. Heart disease is still the number one cause of death in the U.S., and in 2011 claimed 596,339 lives.[177] It would have been 1.9 million deaths if the total had been at the 1950 rate.

We have shown that trans fats interfere with the body's mechanisms to keep blood flowing, a key factor in heart disease. While the 1968 reduction in the trans fat content of margarine and shortening have contributed to the reduction in heart disease mortality, our data suggests that this reduction was not enough and that trans fats from partially hydrogenated oils should be completely eliminated from the diet. Even processed foods labeled as 0% trans fats often contain hidden trans fat that may contribute to this effect, providing an additional reason to support diets that emphasize whole foods over processed foods to reduce the risk of heart disease. I am sure you agree with me now that banning trans fats will help reduce heart disease.

Fat Fried Food

There are problems with deep fat fried food that affect our nutrition. These problems occur because of chemical alterations in the fat that happen as a consequence of deep fat frying food. This frying process is as follows:

1. Food picks up oxygen from the air during frying that negatively alters the fat composition.
2. The foods fried in these fats pick up those altered fats.
3. These altered foods have a direct and negative influence on the nutritional value of the fat.

The changes in the fat are dependent on at least four factors:

1. The length of time it was exposed to heat—in commercial operations, the length of time a

food is fried leads to how much fat is absorbed on the "cooked" food item;

2.   The temperature of the fat;

3.   The exact composition of the fat used, such as corn oil, cottonseed oil, soybean oil, beef tallow, or hydrogenated fat, and

4.   What is being fried, e.g., chicken or fish.

The longer the frying fat is heated, the greater the changes in that fat. Feeding animals fats fried at varying lengths of time led to very different outcomes in the health of those animals. Those fed the fats fried the shortest period of time were healthier than those fed the fats fried for the longest times.[178,179] Those fed fats heated at higher temperatures were not as healthy as those fed on fat heated to lower temperatures. Also it was interesting that animals fed on heated margarine did not grow as well as those on fresh margarine and that their plasma cholesterol level increased. Those fed on heated butter oil grew as well as those on fresh butter oil.[180]

Oil from commercial fat fryers was used in a set of experiments that clearly showed that poor nutrition resulted. This is important because used fat from commercial operations is typically collected and fed to animals, such as pigs, to provide energy for rapid growth. When we conducted experiments feeding the commercially used fat for frying to rats, they did not do well. When we added protein to their diets, the effect of the "bad" heated fat was countered because the added protein provided more adequate nutrition.[181]We tried to fortify the diets with adequate vitamins, but that could not counter the growth-depressing effect of the heated oil. A few vitamins, such as riboflavin, helped a bit.[182]

Fish already contain high amounts of polyunsaturated fat that are not present in the fat of chicken or beef. Thus, when fish are fried, the polyunsaturated fat in them can leak into the frying fat causing the fat to be changed more radically into a less healthy version. Chicken and hamburger have less of this polyunsaturated fat and thus are healthier choices to fry. Eating excessive amounts of fried food also slows down digestion. People may get stomachaches as a result. As early as 1946, a link was shown between heated fats and cancer.[183] What we don't know yet is whether heated fats by themselves lead to cancer or whether the heated fat combined with specific foods cause cancer. Animals fed heated fat combined with a known carcinogen developed cancer, whereas those fed fresh fat combined with a known carcinogen, did not. Thus the heated fat was a co-carcinogen.[184]

Commercial frying of food has increased worldwide since our studies on heated fats. In Germany, fat fryers are required by law to test their frying fat for its freshness by a method approved by the German government. In the U.S. a test is also available but its use is not mandatory.

Free Radicals

Free radicals are produced from oxidized linoleic (n-6) and linolenic acid (n-3); they are fragments of unsaturated fatty acids.[185,186] This is especially likely to happen when the essential fatty acids are heated, especially the n-3 variety. All oils change structures when they are heated, but those high in n-3 fatty acids have more problems than those high in n-6. Free radicals provide another reason to avoid fried food. The first sign of fat becoming free radicals is that they are rancid, and they begin to smell "off" and their taste becomes bitter. Roasted peanuts, for example, can become rancid and then shouldn't be eaten.

Free radicals are "bad" since they destroy vitamins A, D, C, and E, thus preventing these vitamins from doing positive things in the body. Free radicals also destroy both the essential fatty acids and the essential amino acids. They oxidize the LDL into something called oxidized low density lipoproteins (oxLDL). These oxLDL are very powerful components in the blood that have been considered since about 1990 as involved in the development of heart disease.[186]

The best way to avoid free radicals is simply not eating fried food nor any foods with oil that smells "off."

CHAPTER 2 : Key Points

- Fats have essential nutrients that can only come from the diet.
- Animal fat, containing both saturated and unsaturated fat, should be eaten since it provides both essential fatty acids.
- Not all fats are created equal; make sure the ones you eat contain the essential fatty acids (n-3 or omega-3 and n-6 or omega-6).
- The amount of fat you eat is important since too much leads to obesity and too little causes other health problems.
- Until all trans fats have been removed from food products, continue to read food labels to avoid any product that contains partially hydrogenated fat in its ingredients list.
- Avoid fried foods; if you do eat them, eat protein with them from sources such as fish, chicken, or hamburger.
- If you fry food yourself, use the fat only twice and refrigerate it between uses.
- Avoid eating between meals so that the body can use its fat in its fasting period.
- Remember it's not the fats alone that lead to health problems; it's also the overabundance of calories often because of too much carbohydrate

(sugar, starch) and fat in the food. In limited quantities, fats are essential to our wellbeing.

CHAPTER 3: All Proteins are <u>Not</u> the Same

Protein seems to be a popular food now, with diets touting high protein consumption. Protein is, of course, an important building block in the body, but it is not the only building block, as we've shown with the previous chapters. And furthermore, protein is made up of a variety of substances, with the result that not all protein sources are equal in value. Here are some of the facts about proteins. Did you know that:

- Protein is essential to a healthy heart and a healthy body.
- Not all protein sources are equal in nutritional value.
- Animal sources of protein including eggs are "better" for you nutritionally since they contain all of the essential amino acids. As with most nutrients and vitamins, both too much and too little protein have detrimental effects on the body.
- Protein cannot be "stocked" up like fat and must be eaten daily.

Protein is the basic nutrient and plays an essential role in carrying cholesterol and preventing heart disease. The human body in its complexity needs dozens of nutritive substances. The one that stands before all others is protein, or proteins, since there is not one but hundreds of kinds of protein.

Here's what protein contributes:

- We are literally made of protein from our bones to our muscles, arteries and veins, skin, hair, and fingernails. Our heart, brain, liver, kidneys, and lungs are built of tissue made of proteins.

- Proteins help carry the oxygen that reddens our blood. In the form of enzymes, proteins digest our food, synthesize essential substances, and break down waste products for elimination.

- When fat and carbohydrates are insufficient, proteins produce the energy we need for life.

- Proteins in combination with a substance called sterols form hormones, which regulate the delicate chemical changes that constantly take place within the body.

- The chromosomes, which pass on our characteristics to our children, include protein in their structure.

- Protein is needed to "carry" fat and cholesterol throughout the body.

To be short on protein is to be lacking in the very substance of life.

Proteins are Building Blocks

Proteins, our most complex substances, are made up of varying combinations of nitrogen-containing amino acids, the building blocks from which proteins are made.[187] There are 20 different amino acids that are important to the body. These 20 combine together in hundreds of intricate chemical patterns to create a variety of complex protein structures. When we eat foods that are sources of protein, such as meat, milk, cheese, eggs, beans, or peas, the digestive system first breaks down the food proteins into their amino acids, and after they are absorbed into the blood, enzymes in the body recombine them into a certain sequence to produce the proteins suited to the body's special needs, such as making red blood cells or building muscles. The body has the ability to make its own "building blocks" out of whatever amino acids are on hand. However, there is one important limitation—some of those amino acids are only available in food. These "raw materials" so to speak must all be present to build the body properly; if they are not, the body, like a building made with shoddy materials, will not stand up over time. Of the 20 amino acids needed for proper construction, eight are called essential amino acids (nine for children) since the body cannot synthesize or make these for itself: histidine, isoleucine, leucine, lysine, methionine + cystine, phenylalanine + tyrosine, threonine, tryptophan, and valine. These essential amino acids must come from our diets.[188] The other twelve can be manufactured within the body or to continue our construction metaphor, they are made "on-site." At different ages, we need different amounts of amino acids for optimal functioning. The next sections look first at how much protein (and amino acids) we need overall, and second at the unequal sources of amino acids in these proteins. Not all protein sources have equal nutritional value.

Amount of Protein Needed Daily

There are two issues in this section—the amounts of the essential amino acids as well as total amount of protein needed. The body requires not only food to supply the nine essential amino acids it cannot make on its own, but also foods in the right amounts to help in the process of using and making those other 12 amino acids within the body.

Table 4: Recommended Daily Allowance (RDA) of the Essential Amino Acids in terms of mg/kg of weight (2.2 lb/kg)[33]

Amino Acid	Infants (<1 year)	Children (1-3y)	Adolescents (12-18y)		Adults (19y+)
			Girls	Boys	
Histidine	32	21	14	15	14
Isoleucine	43	28	19	21	19
Leucine	93	63	44	47	42
Lysine	89	58	40	48	38
Methionine + cysteine*	43	28	19	21	19
Phenylalanine + tyrosine**	84	54	35	38	33
Threonine	49	32	21	22	20
Tryptophan	13	8	5	6	5
Valine	58	37	24	27	4

* Methionine gets converted to cysteine. **Phenylalanine gets converted to tyrosine.

Table 4 presents the nine essential amino acids, as well as the amounts needed according to age, activity level, and health[189].

Figure 3 illustrates this same data graphically. All of the figures contain the essential amino acids numbered as in Table 4.

Figure 3. The recommended daily allowances (RDA) of the nine essential amino acids by age groups in mg/kg of weight[189]

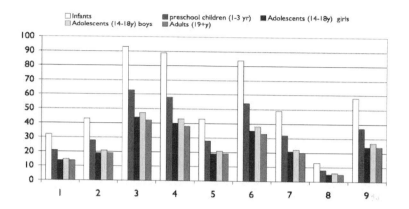

Note how much more infants need of every essential amino acid than adults. Of all the sources of amino acids, the best source is nature's most perfect food—mother's milk.[33] Figure 4 compares the amino acid needs of infants with what is provided in mother's milk. Infants typically consume about one quart of milk per day (or the equivalent of 946 mL). Figure 5 shows that this amount meets the complete daily requirement of protein for an infant weighing about 9 pounds (or 4 kilograms). Infants need more of the essential amino acids than do adults. Refer back to Table 4 and Figure 3 that spell out the amounts needed at all age groups; remember those needed in greatest amounts at all ages are Leucine (#3), Lysine (#4), and Phenylalanine (#6). The bars of the graphs for these three should always be the longest to help ensure adequate amounts of these amino acids. It is interesting to note that the one quart of mother's milk contains the needed mixture in the right amounts of essential amino acids daily required by the infant; note that the bars mirror each other in length. The amino acids that are

69

required in greater amounts appear in greater volume in the mother's milk.

Figure 4. Daily amino acid requirement of an infant compared with the human milk consumption of an infant[33]

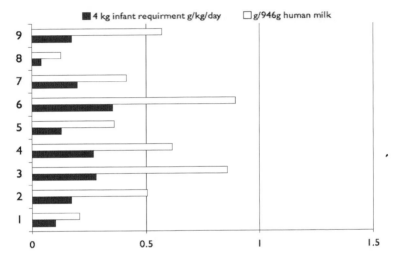

1) Histidine 2) Isoleucine 3) Leucine 4) Lysine 5) Methionine + Cystine 6) Phenylalanine + Tyrosine 7) Threonine 8) Tryptophan 9) Valine g/100g

The next question then concerns how much protein overall do we need each day? The National Research Council of the National Academy of Sciences has established a "Recommended Daily Allowance" (RDA)[189] for protein (see Table 5), but it is important to recognize that no set allowance, based on averages, can speak for the widely differing requirements of every individual.

As with all other nutrients such as vitamins and minerals, the amount of protein required depends on the individual's age, weight, sex, level of activity, total intake of calories, and health. Other considerations may also be important; growing children and teenagers, pregnant women, and persons recovering from illness all need more protein than the "average" person. As shown in Table 5, growing children and teenagers need more protein than adults. A 65-pound child requires about 59 grams of protein per day, more than his or her 180-pound father. Pregnant women and breastfeeding mothers also need additional protein since they are not only maintaining their own bodies but also providing for the growth of their developing child. The pregnant teenager has an even greater need: she has to supply her own fast-growing body while nourishing the fetus developing within her womb. For a pregnant teenage girl of 110 pounds, the protein requirement goes up to about 62.5 grams per day, much higher than for an adolescent of the same age. A pregnant teenager who does not eat enough protein will give birth to an underweight baby who may not survive. The data above is based on both weight and other body requirements, such as pregnancy to predict the amount of protein needed. Since pregnant teenagers generally weigh less than adult women who are pregnant, the result is a lower amount of suggested protein for a pregnant teenager than for the pregnant adult.

Table 5: RDA Suggested Amounts of Pure Protein Needed Daily[189]

Person's characteristics	Amount of "pure" protein needed	
	Grams/day	Ounces/day
Adult male (180 pounds)	47.4	1.67
Adult female (135 lbs)	44.6	1.57
Child (65 lbs)	59	2.08
Pregnant woman (160 lbs)	67	2.36
Adolescent (100 lbs)	39.2	1.38
Pregnant teenager (110 lbs)	62.5	2.20

It is worth pausing to consider that the protein in our body is constantly being destroyed, i.e., it is used up during normal metabolism. A study on the rate at which a protein is "used up" has been carried out in swine.[190] Swine were used because they are the animal closest to us in how food is

71

metabolized. This study indicated that it took 36 hours before the protein was used up. "Used up" in this case means the protein was freed of its nitrogen and no longer furnishing building blocks for body tissue. This study compared feeding pregnant swine every day with feeding pregnant swine with the same amount of food, but every three days. The pregnant swine fed every day gave birth to heavier and healthier piglets than those fed every third day.

As far as I'm aware, studies on humans to date do not cover this "transit time" for proteins. However, I believe the protein metabolism works the same way in people. This means that eating a hamburger or a steak on Sunday will not still supply an adequate amount of essential amino acids on Tuesday, even though on Sunday all the essential amino acids were there. Even more problematical is eating soy-based cheese pizza five times a week because it is convenient. This food is likely missing an essential amino acid, as shown in the next section. Both soy products and wheat flour are considered "incomplete" proteins since they do not have all of the essential amino acids in adequate amounts. The body needs all the amino acids to make cells, such as those in muscles.

As discussed in Chapter 1, cholesterol is carried in the blood by lipoproteins. Lipoproteins include (1) apoproteins, combinations of essential and nonessential amino acids in varying amounts; (2) phospholipid, a fat and water-soluble complex; and (3) fat. These apoprotein carriers must be carefully constructed by the body out of the correct combination of essential and nonessential amino acids. These carriers cannot be made properly if one of the essential amino acids is missing—another reason not to short yourself on the essential amino acids. The important role of apoproteins in transporting cholesterol in the blood has been documented[23] and there has been an immense amount of research tying differences in apoproteins to a possible cause for heart disease.

Not only must all the essential amino acids be present, they must also be present in the right amounts to carry cholesterol. Chickens have a similar metabolism to human beings and are often used in scientific experiments. A study[191] in which one-week-old chicks were fed various combinations of both essential and non-essential amino acids showed that the lowest cholesterol level was always in the chicks fed the required essential amino acids in the correct amount. Whenever an essential amino acid was missing or even a non-essential amino acid was fed in excess, the cholesterol level increased. This may also happen in people eating unbalanced amino acid diets, although to verify such a study today is not possible in the human population. It has been assumed that Americans consume more than an adequate amount of protein, although we do not know if this happens every day and in the right amounts. An adequate amount of essential amino acids must be supplied every day of the week for optimum nutrition.

For the body to function properly we also need to take in considerably more protein than the amount we use. The rate of protein use or destruction in the body is about 0.33 grams of protein for each kilogram (2.2 pounds) of body weight per day.[23](To help put this in context for those not metrically inclined, 100 grams = 3.53 ounces and 1 ounce = 28.5 grams. A 75 kg./165 pound person would use up 24.75 grams or slightly less than one ounce per day of protein.) The RDA amounts in Table 6 refer to the protein itself, not the food it is found in. As we discussed, foods containing protein also contain other nutrients.

Unequal Protein Sources

The goal in any diet is to eat an adequate amount of each essential amino acid to satisfy the recommended daily requirement.[189] However, just because various foods contain protein does not mean that those proteins are all equal in nutritional value. Different proteins contain differing amounts of those essential amino acids, and some, when eaten in a regular serving, do not contain enough to satisfy the body's requirements. In this section, we'll show some common foods and their essential amino acids contents. You'll see why some sources, such as meat and eggs, are called "complete" proteins since they contain all of the nine essential amino acids. "Incomplete" proteins, such as in tofu made from soybeans, are labeled that way since they do not have large enough amounts of all the essential amino acids.

We'll be looking at a variety of complete and incomplete proteins in Figures 4 to 17. The white bars on each of the figures indicate the food source that contains the greatest amount of the nine essential amino acids in grams out of 100 grams. In looking at the figures, keep in mind that the longer the bar, the higher the amount of that amino acid. A protein source that contains two grams of an essential amino acid is more nutritious than one that contains one gram of an essential amino acid. These graphs were constructed from the percentage of essential amino acids in food items listed by the USDA Nutrient Data Laboratory.[187] Each of the essential amino acids is numbered in the figures for easy reference.

Figure 5. Essential amino acids in human milk compared to one egg[187]

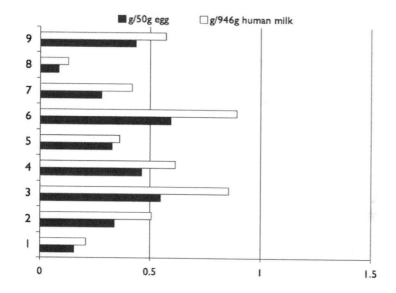

We've discussed how mother's milk is nature's most perfect food, and Figure 6 shows the egg to be in second place because its amino acid contents mimic the levels in mother's milk. The egg contains less fat per gram than meat, and also it is inexpensive and readily available. If you doubled the portion to two whole eggs, these would contain even more of the essential amino acids than one quart of human milk, although our data here is based only on a one-egg comparison.

Figure 6 compares some common sources of animal proteins along with a common vegetarian source, tofu. Pork provides the most amino acids of all of these sources, and tofu, the least. It is a myth that eating tofu provides the same nutritional value as eating pork, beef, salmon, or chicken. Tofu is especially deficient in methionine and tryptophan. As you can see, different proteins contain different amounts of amino acids.

Figure 6. Comparison of the essential amino acids of pork, beef, chicken, salmon and tofu[187]

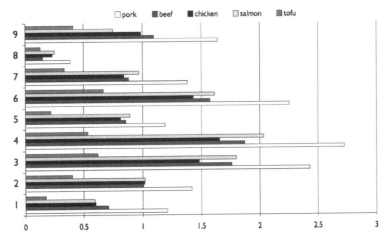

1) Histidine 2) Isoleucine 3) Leucine 4) Lysine 5) Methionine + Cystine6) Phenylalanine + Tyrosine 7) Threonine 8) Tryptophan 9) Valine g/100g

As shown in Figure 7, various parts of the egg contain different portions of the essential amino acids. Many people just eat one part of the egg, the white or the yolk, for ostensibly better health. If you just eat the white of the egg, you'll get less nutritional value than available from either the yolk or the whole egg. The white contains only protein, but no vitamins or minerals. If you eat just the yolk, you'll get less of one essential amino acid, tryptophan (#8), than from either the white or the whole egg. The egg yolk also contains vitamins, minerals, and a little fat. It's best to eat the whole egg for maximum nutritional value.

Figure 7. Comparison of equal amounts of egg white, egg yolk and whole eggs[187]

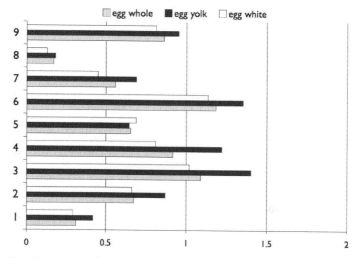

To illustrate the essential amino acid content of a number of foods, we've created additional figures to readily show which protein sources have the largest amount g/100g of essential amino acids. First, we focus on wheat, an incomplete protein. The amino acid amount in the whole wheat kernel is greater than in wheat flour, whole wheat bread, and white bread. Wheat is lower in tryptophan (#8 in the graph) than is needed. The longest bars in Figure 8 indicate that the wheat kernel contains more of the nine amino acids than wheat flour, and that whole wheat bread contains more of the amino acids than white bread. Most of us eat wheat in bread, either of the whole wheat or the white bread variety, not a whole wheat kernel. Figure 8 illustrates the point that the grains we currently eat do not furnish enough protein to be a major source of protein in our diet.

Figure 8. Amino acids in whole wheat kernel, wheat flour, whole wheat bread and white bread[187]

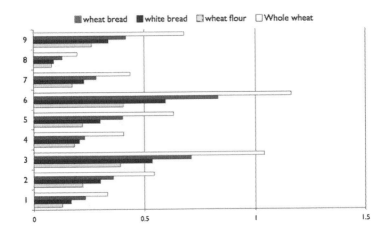

1) Histidine 2) Isoleucine 3) Leucine 4) Lysine 5) Methionine + Cystine 6) Phenylalanine + Tyrosine 7) Threonine 8) Tryptophan 9) Valine g/100g

Figure 9 illustrates our concern with the lower amounts of essential amino acids in grains versus animal products. Here the comparison is between the whole wheat kernel, a form most of us do not eat, and one egg. Note how much more of the amino acids are in the complete protein, egg, versus the incomplete one of wheat. Comparing protein sources and their amino acid contents can get somewhat complicated, as shown in Figures 9-16.

Figure 9. The amount of essential amino acids in 100g of whole wheat compared to 100g of egg[187]

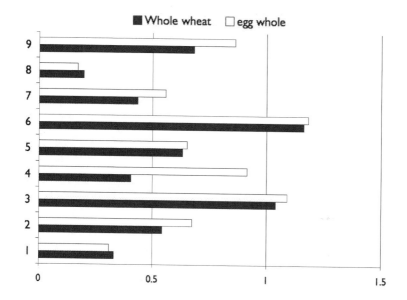

The amounts of amino acids in 100g of navy beans and corn are compared in Figure 10. As shown, both are low in tryptophan (#8) and methionine (#5). Corn is also low in lysine (#4). Corn contains more of the essential amino acids than beans in five of the nine, but beans can help balance the corn in the other four areas. That is why beans and corn are often served together in the Mexican diet, for example. Those who eat only vegetable proteins need to pay careful attention to the amount of amino acids in each source to make sure they have enough overall.

Figure 10. The essential amino acids in navy beans compared to corn[187]

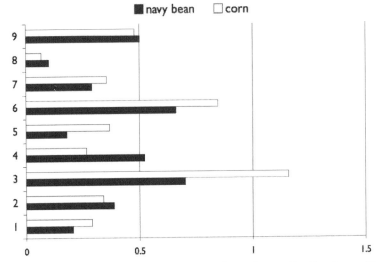

1) Histidine 2) Isoleucine 3) Leucine 4) Lysine 5) Methionine + Cystine 6) Phenylalanine + Tyrosine 7) Threonine 8) Tryptophan 9) Valine g/100g

Figure 11 compares two incomplete proteins—navy beans and wheat bread—with a complete protein, in this case chicken. You can clearly see the superiority of chicken in providing the essential amino acids. Yet the first two items, wheat bread and navy beans, are those the USDA recommends as sources of amino acids to substitute for meat, milk, and eggs. This figure illustrates why this is inadequate advice. It is a myth to say all protein sources are equal.

Figure 11. The essential amino acids in chicken, wheat bread and navy beans[187]

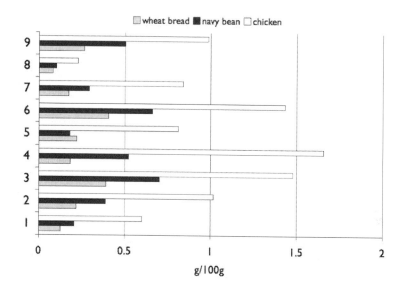

The "incomplete" proteins from grains and vegetable sources—corn, rice, peas, beans, nuts, and sesame seeds—contain all nine essential amino acids but not in the same amounts and not in adequate amounts as in eggs, dairy products, and meat. However, as we showed above, it is possible to obtain the nine essential amino acids, piecemeal fashion, by eating several kinds of vegetable proteins like corn, beans, and soybeans at the same time. Also if you eat an extra large amount of the incomplete proteins, you can get 100% of what you need. However, you may not have a large enough stomach to eat anything else and thus miss out on other important nutrients!

The amino acid content of various dairy products and soymilk, a substitute used for milk, are compared in Figure 12. Cheese products, both American (cheddar) cheese and cottage cheese, contain all of the essential amino acids in large quantities. Every type of cow's milk from whole milk to skim milk has the same amounts of amino acids; the only difference is in the fat and water content of the dairy product itself. Milk is used to make cheese; in fact it takes about five quarts of whole milk to make one pound of cheddar cheese. Since cheese is so "concentrated" and has far less water than milk, it contains greater amounts of amino acids ounce for ounce (or gram for gram in this case) than milk. Cheese also contains ten times more fat than whole milk, as well as ten times more protein. The fat provides the flavor in cheese. Comparing milk and soymilk, it is clear that soymilk has less of the essential amino acids overall, and is especially low in methionine (#5) and tryptophan (#8). It is not a complete substitute for cow's milk, yet it costs more. Milk and milk products provide both protein and calcium that are needed by people at all ages. Many adults consider milk just for infants. However, the increasing amount of osteoporosis in the bones of both men and women indicates that many Americans don't drink enough milk or eat enough dairy products to retain normal bone function throughout the lifespan.

Figure 12. Comparison of Dairy Products and Soy Milk[187]

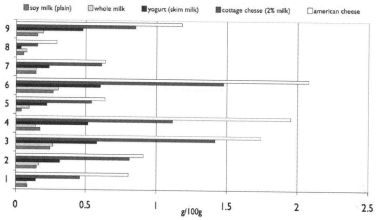

1) Histidine 2) Isoleucine 3) Leucine 4) Lysine 5) Methionine + Cystine6) Phenylalanine + Tyrosine 7) Threonine 8) Tryptophan 9) Valine g/100g

Nuts (such as walnuts, pecans, and almonds) like vegetable proteins can serve well as supplementary protein sources even though they are an incomplete protein. Nuts also provide something additional to the nutritional picture, polyunsaturated fatty acids which were explained in Chapter 2. Figure 13 shows the essential amino acids in pecans, sesame seeds, and peanuts. Pecans contain lesser amounts of eight amino acids than peanuts or sesame seed. Peanuts have the highest amounts of six of the amino acids. Overall, nuts come up short when compared to animal sources of protein, and furthermore they can contribute too much fat to the diet.

Figure 13. Comparison of essential amino acids in nuts and seeds[187]

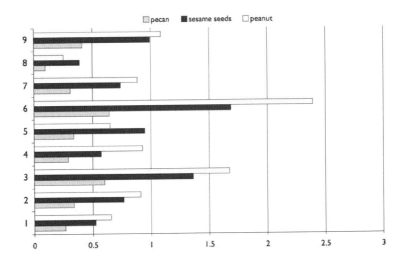

Continuing to look at grains as a source of protein leads to the next comparison, that of several kinds of starches. Figure 14 compares the amino acid contents of white rice, wild rice, and pasta. None contain much protein. Pasta is made from wheat flour, which has less protein due to its milling process. White rice has some of its protein removed in the milling process as well. Wild rice is not polished so more of its protein remains, although in some instances, pasta is a better source of several amino acids than the other two. However, none of them are good sources of the essential amino acids.

Figure 14. The amino acids of white rice, wild rice and pasta[187]

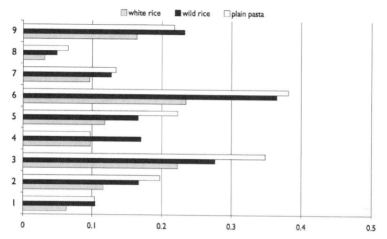

1) Histidine 2) Isoleucine 3) Leucine 4) Lysine 5) Methionine + Cystine 6) Phenylalanine + Tyrosine 7) Threonine 8) Tryptophan 9) Valine g/100g

Now let's compare some popular foods, hamburgers and pizzas. Figure 15 illustrates that a hamburger has more nutritional value than a cheese pizza. While pizza contains 9-12% of fat, hamburger contains 9-18% of fat. However, hamburger has more than twice as much protein as pizza (25% and 11% respectively).

Figure 15. Amino Acid comparisons[187]

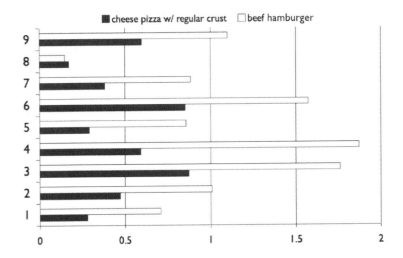

When the "right" two incomplete proteins are combined, the value of their amino acids almost equals that of a complete protein. For example, a combination of 50g beans with 50g of corn is better than 100 grams of eggs but not quite as good as beef, as shown in Figure 16.

Figure 16. Comparison of 50g beans+50g of corn with 100g of beef or 100g whole egg[187]

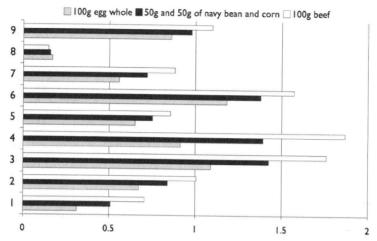

1) Histidine 2) Isoleucine 3) Leucine 4) Lysine 5) Methionine + Cystine 6) Phenylalanine + Tyrosine 7) Threonine 8) Tryptophan 9) Valine g/100g

It is interesting to note that pet foods for dogs and cats are carefully formulated to include the right amounts of essential amino acids. My colleagues in the College of Veterinary Medicine tell me that the coronary arteries of pet dogs and cats contain very little atherosclerosis. Unfortunately, people do not have such a carefully formulated diet, although we have all of the essential food components supplied by a food industry with products now readily available in every developed country in the world.

As we've shown above, "complete" proteins, those that contain all of the "essential" amino acids, are found in significant amounts only in meat, milk, and eggs. Furthermore, these amino acids exist in those products in the proportions that resemble very closely the proportions needed by the human body. Thus it is more nutritionally efficient to get the essential amino acids from animal products, using vegetable and nut proteins as valuable supplements. You need all the essential amino acids, so paying attention to which ones are missing in which foods is important to overall dietary health, especially if you are a vegetarian or a vegan. This, however, is not easy to do.

Although all processed food contains the amount of protein, fat, and carbohydrate on the label, I know of none that also lists the amount of essential amino acids on the label. Such information would be useful to vegetarians to calculate a daily intake of all of the essential amino acids in adequate amounts. The information is available from the USDA Nutrient Data Laboratory[187] that includes the percentage of protein, fat, minerals, vitamins, and amino acid content in gram/100gram of many foods (www.nal.usda.gov/fnic/foodcomp/search). These data must have taken many hours to collect, but is presently unavailable to the average consumer. If it were readily available, one could plan meals that would waste less protein and assure the daily intake of all of the essential amino acids. This could have the added benefit of decreasing overall caloric intake.

Eggs

Because eggs have been so maligned in nutritional recommendations, a whole section needs to be devoted to this food source. Eggs are the most nutritious and the least expensive protein source in the grocery store. Remember, eggs are a "complete" protein, that is, they contain all the amino acids your body needs each day. One egg provides 68 calories and about 11% of your daily protein requirement. Eggs contain a variety of important nutrients including almost every vitamin, mineral and natural antioxidant that your body needs. Those nutrients are enough to feed a growing chick so that it hatches healthy, but not enough for you to meet your daily requirement! Studies at many major universities in the U.S. and abroad attest to the egg as an excellent source of protein. Many in the forefront of anti-aging research believe that moderate egg consumption of one per day should be an integral part of a complete anti-aging diet.[192]

Because eggs are high in natural cholesterol (210-220 mg of cholesterol per egg), there has been a concern that eating an egg would raise one's cholesterol level to unhealthy levels.[193] Restricting egg consumption became a key component in many health-related diets; this is actually a misguided recommendation since this has not been shown to be the case.[194] Eating an egg raises the total cholesterol score only 2-3 mg/dl on well balanced diets. In healthy young men and women, even two eggs a day had little effect on total cholesterol levels.[195] In a recent study, elderly subjects (more than 60 years old) were assigned to one of two dietary groups: one group ate three eggs per day and the other ate the same amount in egg substitutes for a one-month period.[192] The result of this study was a significant increase in both LDL and HDL cholesterol for those who ate eggs, but the ratio between the two was not affected significantly. In other words, if the LDL went up, the HDL did too, thus counteracting the effect of the higher LDL. The study concluded that dietary cholesterol provided by eggs does not increase the risk for heart disease in an elderly population.

There have been a number of studies conducted looking at egg consumption and health risks. One at Harvard University included an eight to fourteen year follow-up study of approximately 38,000 men and 80,000 women.[196] There was no statistically significant difference in risk for heart attacks and strokes among people who ate eggs less than once a week compared with those who ate more than one egg a day. Other studies in a variety of settings found no evidence that eating up to an egg per day led to heart attacks or strokes.[197] The Framingham study[198] has investigated the effect of environmental factors and what people ate on the development of coronary heart disease since 1949. No relationship between egg intake and coronary heart disease incidence was found. Recently, evidence has been accumulating to suggest that eating foods containing cholesterol is less relevant to cardiovascular risk than eating foods containing fat.[199] For example, people who ate either oats or eggs daily for six weeks ended up with similar cholesterol levels and similar weights. Hospitalized patients eating eggs and tested at intervals of five hours to 54 days found no significant differences in cholesterol levels.[200] In a diet that contains at least 25 grams of fiber, only a few milligrams of cholesterol in an egg were absorbed from the intestinal tract.[201]

So how did eggs end up being so maligned? In 1975, the Federal Trade Commission (FTC) held hearings on eggs after egg producers had advertised that eggs do not cause heart attacks.[202,203] Only two witnesses testified in favor of the egg; I was one. The other was Dr. DeBakey; apparently because he was a (famous heart) surgeon, not a cardiologist, he also did not hold sway. All the other witnesses testified that eggs contained cholesterol, and cholesterol causes heart disease, therefore do not eat eggs. The anti-egg scientists who testified based their testimony on two significant experiments. One involved feeding of cholesterol containing food, including eggs, to rabbits. The rabbits did indeed have much higher cholesterol levels in their blood and they developed atherosclerosis.[25] What wasn't said was that rabbits do not ever eat cholesterol as part of their normal diet. We would expect rabbits to not do well with such a diet, and indeed that was the case. The second major experiment was done by feeding egg yolks (not whole eggs) to Indians in Northern Mexico.[188,189] Their cholesterol levels went up 40 points. What should have been done was feeding whole eggs instead of just the yolk because the body needs the extra protein in the egg white to help metabolize the cholesterol.[190] (Part of the moral here is to eat both the yolk and the white of the egg!) The studies at that time on the pro-egg side were not compelling enough to counteract these two flawed experiments. The flaws in these studies were never brought to light, and probably were even unknown to the researchers at the time. We now know that humans have a defense system of enzymes that metabolize dietary sources of cholesterol and have a means of controlling the amount of cholesterol synthesized by the liver.[11,12] Most experimental feeding studies have used an excess of dietary cholesterol that overwhelmed the defense system and led to false conclusions.

Egg producers lost and could no longer advertise eggs by saying they did not cause heart attacks. This actually led to a greater loss for the American population who were discouraged from eating an excellent and inexpensive food item that could help counteract the high intake of fat and sugar in the American diet, which had been steadily increasing since 1950. A later ad campaign for eggs used the phrase, "the incredible, edible egg."[204] That certainly is true.

Substituting Plant for Animal Proteins

Much of the world population tries to meet their need for protein with plant sources. Indeed even in the U.S., grains and cereals are a large part of the recommended diet for protein, vitamins, and minerals. The possible effects of moving away from animal protein to those of plant sources should be considered.

In 1971, Frances Moore Lappe[205] published her book, Diet for a Small Planet, a book that claimed to have started a revolution for the way Americans eat. This book was revised as a second edition 20 years later. The book advocated the use of cereals and legumes rather than animal protein products for the American diet because it was assumed that the cereal grains fed to animals could be more effectively used to feed the human population. The book had an impact on diet recommendation of the American Heart Association and the USDA because grains and legumes do not contain cholesterol and therefore are assumed to be less likely to cause heart disease than the cholesterol in animal food products such as meat, cheese, and eggs.

Lappe was aware that meat, cheese, and eggs had a greater biological value than either cereals or legumes because animal food products had an essential amino acid mix that was more complete than either the amino acid content in the protein of cereals or legumes. She reasoned that combinations of vegetable and grain sources such as wheat and beans or soybeans would provide a sufficient supply of essential amino acids. There are three flaws in Lappe's thinking. One is the very nature of plant proteins and their manufacturing process. Processed cereals are deficient in minerals and vitamins. Furthermore plant proteins are incomplete proteins and need to be eaten in combination. The second flaw is the lack of available land to grow plant proteins. Grassland that is used to graze animals cannot be converted easily into land to grow plant proteins nor should it be so converted. Third, animals actually function very effectively to convert plants that people could not live on, such as grass, into animal protein that people can digest.

Dr. Marion Nestle, a professor of Nutrition at New York University and author of a book entitled What to Eat [206] adds organic food as an aspect to the nutritional evaluation of vegetable and fruit sources. The assumption is that vegetables and fruits that are grown under such conditions are "fresher," have more taste appeal and possibly more nutritional value, and do not have the negative effects of pesticides. Organic foods are grown with organic rather than mineral sources of fertilizer and with USDA certified pesticides and herbicides; they are not pesticide-free. They are also grown with organic fertilizer (manure) rather than mineral sources of fertilizer containing nitrogen, phosphate, and potassium. A side benefit of this organic fertilizer is that the nutrients from the manure of animal operations now can be used to grow plants, rather than end up as run-off into rivers and ponds. That run-off with its excess of nutrients often contributes to plant growth in the water, such as algae blooms.

It would be impossible for all crops to be grown organically or by methods used in the 1950s and still feed the world. In 1950 an acre of land in central Illinois yielded 80 bushels of corn; that same acre can yield as much as 250 bushels of corn today.[207] Two factors make this possible—better seed and synthetic fertilizer. Ammonia is synthesized from natural gas and is the nitrogen source needed to grow crops. Crops grown with synthetic fertilizer have the same nutritive value as those grown organically. Organically grown foods cost more money but if you gain satisfaction eating them, by all means do so. When it comes to health issues, the increased expense of organic food is only a small part of the total amount of money spent for better health.

Plant Proteins

If we decrease our animal protein consumption, we would have to rely more on protein-containing plants. Grains and cereals are a large part of the recommended diet for protein, vitamins, and minerals. Another plant source of additional protein are the legumes—peas and beans, with soybeans taking an increasingly important role. In recent years it has become technologically feasible to isolate good quality protein from soybeans and other legume plants, and many experts have predicted that a major source of our protein may someday come from this source. Yet, at present, most consumers have demonstrated little inclination to buy and eat the products made from such processed vegetable proteins. We can increase our consumption of vegetable proteins in the form of supplements to our bread and other baked goods. Some products have been developed as substitutes for meat, such as soy hamburgers and soybean milk, which cost more than products from cows. Few people, so far, have shown that they are willing to pay higher prices for protein foods that may be less tasty than real meat, milk, and eggs.

Both economically and nutritionally, the proposed redirection of legume and cereal protein from animals to people is not a serious issue. The protein from soybeans, alfalfa, corn, wheat, and rice and their various byproducts is not actually lost. Ninety percent of the protein from legumes in the U.S., like the 85% of soybeans and its byproducts, is being marketed as feed for livestock. It is fed to livestock and chickens and reaches us eventually in the form of meat, milk, and eggs.

We need to bear in mind that nearly all foods have to be industrially processed in some way before they can be eaten by the consumer. Cereals like wheat, corn, and rice have to be milled, and soybeans require extensive, costly high-technology processing. The cattle, pigs, and chickens that are fed the majority of the grains and legumes produced in this country actually serve us as complex, natural "refining plants." Animals fed on the grains and legumes and on pasture grasses, convert them for us into high-protein foods "fortified" by nature with a variety of essential vitamins and minerals.

Vegetable proteins make valuable contributions as part of a balanced diet. However, we need to realize that in terms of protein quality and calories, vegetable proteins are not nearly the bargain they at first seem since they do not contain sufficient amounts of the essential amino acids. Only those who take the time to carefully balance the amino acids in the various plant proteins will have a healthy diet. Vegetable proteins are extremely useful in a mixed diet that also includes protein from meat, milk, and eggs, but alone, or as the major source, plant proteins fall short for most people.

This basic difference in quality also means that it can be risky to try to replace animal protein with vegetable protein "substitutes," even when they are disguised through processing to resemble the real thing. For example, when "Egg Beaters" first came on the market, we tested them on rats.[208] Rats were the best animals to use for the experiments we were conducting at the time. "Egg Beaters" were advertised as egg substitute that were just as nutritious as farm fresh eggs and even better because they contained no cholesterol. We fed one group of rats on whole eggs and another on "Egg Beaters." The egg-fed rats grew strong and healthy, while the rats fed "Egg Beaters" became underweight and scrawny, lost their hair, and died after only a few weeks. The "Egg Beaters" formula was deficient in an essential vitamin, pantothenic acid. According to the listing of ingredients now on the box, that vitamin has been added and corn oil deleted from the original formula. The present formula, therefore, contains neither fat nor cholesterol, and now has less vitamin E than the original formula. This could lead to other problems. Today, a carton of "Egg Beaters" still costs twice as much as a dozen eggs and still does not equal the nutritional value of the real thing.

A comparison of the biological value of substitutes for eggs, meat, and milk as protein sources brings up a concern for the consumer. Claims are made or implied that cholesterol-free substitutes will lower cholesterol levels in the blood with no clinical tests by the producers having been made as proof of its total nutritional value. The Food and Drug Administration has jurisdiction over ingredients used. The Federal Trade Commission has jurisdiction over advertising claims. This leaves a gray area as to whose responsibility it is to see that claims or implications are accurate.

Plant Protein and Agriculture

If we increase our consumption of plant proteins, we would need to increase the acreage devoted to raising plants, but some problems of a practical nature in the way agriculture currently is practiced would occur. The limits of agriculture should be taken into consideration in diet recommendations.[209] Agriculture is defined as the cultivation of land as in raising crops, husbandry, and tillage farming. Unfortunately, only about 20% of the land in the U.S. can be cultivated for crops, but 26% can be used to pasture livestock.[210] Half of the cropland is used to grow feed for livestock. In realistic terms, any major effort to supply additional plant protein for human consumption in the U.S. would require the dismantling of the nation's agricultural industry, since most of American agriculture is directly or indirectly involved in producing livestock either through direct grazing on grasslands or by growing feed on cultivated land.

Critics of our country's agricultural system persistently argue that instead of continuing to use our valuable farmland to grow feeds for animals, we should follow the example of the Chinese and concentrate on growing vegetable protein to be consumed directly by humans. The claim is often repeated that each pound of beef we eat costs four pounds of grain that should be going to feed people. By turning the land to the production of food crops for direct human consumption the argument goes, we would cut our intake of animal fat and cholesterol and at the same time increase the total food supply by eliminating the inefficiency inherent in animal production. This view, as agro-economists have often shown, overlooks a number of important considerations, quite apart from the questionable willingness on the part of the public to eat wheat, corn, and soybeans in the place of meat, milk, and eggs. The simple truth is that the animal-oriented agricultural system as it has evolved over two centuries in America makes a more efficient use of available land to provide essential, high-quality protein, with fewer surplus calories, and at a lower cost, than any other system that has presently been devised.

In the U.S., a large area of the West is grassland that can only be used to feed animals. Not enough water is available to grow crops. Grazing animals can maximize efficiency in the production of nutrients. Feeder cattle are raised on land that is not fit for wheat, corn, or soybeans. U.S. grasslands are either fertilized or laced with alfalfa or clover to provide increased forage yields. Soybeans and corn that cannot directly be used for human consumption get turned into a by-product used in animal rations in both the U.S. and Northern Europe. Corn is also being used to make ethanol. There is not a surplus of these soybean and corn residues.

Animal agriculture is huge the world over. China and Vietnam account for more than half the pigs produced worldwide. China and Brazil account for over 25% of poultry exports. Brazil, has become the world's largest meat and soybean exporter. In a world of rapidly increasing population and a potentially shrinking food supply, animal food products are presently an asset to adequate nutrition. Animals are converters of inedible proteins to edible ones. Animals can carry on this operation more economically than have food scientists to date. The ingredients on the label of the bags of animal rations include mill wastes, refined waste from soybean oil production, synthetic amino acids, and discarded fat from commercial fat fryers, all ingredients impossible for people to eat as is. One should think of animals as "screening and processing devices" which provide acceptable sources of nutrients.

The rapid expansion in urban development is almost all at the expense of cultivated and grazing land. Better urban planning could save much of this land. Further expansion of land for cultivation in some countries is being carried out but this may be at the expense of the environment. Countries such as India, China, or the U.S. are unlikely to convert land back to cultivation, so planning now may be the key to prevent this land from being turned into cities and removed from its potential in creating edible products.

Usability of the Protein We Eat

Nearly equal in importance to the completeness, or quality, of the protein we eat is how efficiently and completely the body can use it. Not only do we need all the eight (nine for children) essential amino acids in our diet, we also need them in our body in just the right proportions and at the same time. It does little good taking in a few of the essential amino acids one day and getting the others later in the week. The body simply cannot make effective use of them unless it has them all together at one time. Missing one of the essential amino acids is almost like trying to read a novel in which every ninth page is missing, except that our imaginations can fill in the plot line whereas our bodies cannot fill in the missing amino acid. Moreover, even if all the essential amino acids are present, too little of one can limit the body's effective use of the others.

Table 6: The Biological Value "The Net Protein Utilization of Food[23]

Food	NPU	Amount needed daily if a single food source
Eggs	94%	6 1/2 eggs
Milk	86%	5 1/2 cups milk
Swiss or cheddar cheese	82%	5 ounces
Beefsteak	75%	6.6 ounces
Soybeans	66%	2 cups
Peanuts	56%	2 cups
Whole wheat	53%	36 slides of whole wheat bread
Dried beans and peas	34%	7.2 cups beans

The usability of various protein foods can be expressed in terms of digestibility and biological value.[23] Digestibility simply refers to the percentage of the protein in the given food that the body can absorb. Biological value represents the percentage of the absorbed protein that the body can actually put to work building cells for growth and maintenance. If we multiply digestibility and biological value, we get a measuring index known by nutritionists as Net Protein Utilization (NPU), which stands for the total percentage of the protein that the body can actually use.[23] Without exception, animal proteins have a higher NPU than vegetable proteins. See Table 6.

Net protein utilization tells us, among other things, that when we include animal protein in our diet, we can satisfy our daily protein requirements with smaller amounts of food than if we rely on vegetable products alone. Remember that even if you got your NPU from dried peas or navy beans, you would still be getting an incomplete, low-quality protein, deficient in the essential amino acids the body needs.[62] In terms of its quality and its accessibility to the body, the animal protein in meat, milk, and especially

99

eggs goes further in meeting our needs than protein from plants.

Balance of Protein and Calories

Proteins need to be consumed in the right proportion to fats consumed, and the proteins need to be complete, that is containing all nine essential amino acids. Studies with chickens tell us more about proteins, fat, and cholesterol. In one study,[9] we varied the fat-to-protein ratio in the diet. When the amount of protein in the diet was increased compared to the amount of fat in the diet, the cholesterol level in the chicken's blood dropped, and they had less fat on their bodies. The type of fat consumed made no difference. A "hard" fat such as beef tallow gave results similar to a "soft" fat such as corn oil.[212,213] Translating this to people means that if you're going to eat lots of fat of any kind, make sure you eat enough protein to lessen that increase in cholesterol and a weight gain. Keep in mind, however, that this is not the perfect diet because too many calories of anything, including protein, lead to weight gain.

As stated earlier, one way of monitoring the level of protein-to-fat is through the E/P ratio (energy/protein) of a food item or diet.[9] Energy here is measured in calories which are really units representing the energy-producing potential of a food. The E/P ratio is calculated by dividing the total calories in the food item or diet by its protein content. For example, white bread has an E/P ratio of 32 (275 calories divided by 8.5% of protein.) It is possible to label a food item for its energy content (E/P ratio) and thus add information to present food labeling. This ratio can be a measure of "empty calories," that is foods likely to contribute to obesity, but without the nutrients required for good health. Low E/P ratios are good and high E/P ratios, bad, for our diets; thus an E/P ratio of 12 is good, and one of 65 is bad. As you can see from Table 8, fish products, meats, milk, and eggs have a low E/P ratio; candy bars, doughnuts, cookies, and pies have a high energy to protein ratio. The E/P ratio of a meal can be drastically changed by an increase of a single food item such as a doughnut or by the deletion of a food item such as an egg.

Table 7: Comparison of Energy-Protein Ratio of Various Foods [2]

Food	E/P Ratio	Food	E/P Ratio
Shrimp	5	Cheddar Cheese	16
Cottage Cheese	5	Whole Milk	20
Halibut	6	High Protein Bread	21
Lean Beef	10	Oatmeal	28
Skim Milk	10	White Bread	32
Whole Eggs	12	Candy Bar (with nuts)	54
Broccoli	13	Doughnuts	65
Wheat Germ	15	Cookies	73
Fresh Peas	15	Pie Crust	92

Energy Protein ratio = total calories in 100 g/percent protein

We've explained how the balance between protein and calories is measured. Now we need to look at why this balance is important. The physiological reasons for needing a certain balance of protein and calories are complex; in general they have to do with the fact that it is the proteins that carry the fat, or lipids, in the blood. As previously stated, any excess calories we take in are converted into fat in our bodies, and we need additional protein to cope with it. It is a vast oversimplification, but we might think of protein as a kind of "fat-antidote." However, too many calories from any source overwhelm the system so protein no longer can work as an antidote and the antidote analogy breaks down. The total caloric intake is the problem, not just the fat to protein ratio. Eventually that extra fat is deposited in various places in our bodies.

Because protein is such an essential building block and it has that fat-antidote link, some diet specialists have suggested making it the key food to consume. This is not a good idea nutritionally. When no other nutrients are available, the body has only protein to use for energy. In order for protein to be converted to calories, the kidneys have to remove nitrogen from the amino acids to convert it into a usable form of energy. This process is called deamonization. It overworks the kidneys, which can have some long-lasting, negative effects. An illustration of this comes from some early explorers in the U.S. who died after consuming a diet of rabbits. Rabbit meat is very lean and very high in protein. These early explorers had what was called "rabbit-starvation," since they relied on rabbits for their food.[33] Without other nutrients, their bodies could not cope with the protein. Even Lewis and Clarke noted the effects of too much protein in the diet. However, when explorers ate what was called "pemmican," they survived; pemmican contains both protein and fat. Today, a diet overloaded with protein also taxes the kidney. In other words, good diets must include a variety of nutrients.

Protein Deficiency

Protein deficiency is a serious matter. Growing children, especially, need large amounts of protein and are particularly sensitive to its quality. If they do not get enough of the right kind, their general growth and development suffers—their minds as well as their bodies. In the unborn child and young infant, too little protein means that the cells do not form in sufficient numbers, and the cells that are formed are smaller in size. The child's growth is stunted, and no amount of protein consumed later in life can repair the damage. Protein-deficient infants face a lifetime of being smaller, weaker, and less vital—physically, mentally, and emotionally—than they need to be. Protein deficiency can also be lethal. Children studied in hunger-torn Bangladesh in 1970-71 who were protein-deficient had a death rate 4.5 times higher than better-nourished children in the same locality. Increases in protein can make a dramatic difference in the average physical development in whole populations. In Japan, over the period 1900-1955 when the national consumption of animal protein was increasing, sons grew two inches taller than their fathers, and daughters matured two years earlier than their mothers.[23]

Protein is not only important for growth, but also in the prevention of heart disease. Protein carries the fat throughout the body. If it is deficient, that fat gets deposited on the body, rather than whisked through it. However, if there is too much fat, even the protein cannot handle it and it still gets deposited. It's been shown that people in lower income brackets even in industrialized nations have more heart disease than those in higher brackets; this may be due to the former eating less protein in relationship to the amount of fat consumed.

CHAPTER 3 : Key Points

- High quality protein must be part of any diet because of its overwhelming importance to physical and mental growth and wellbeing.

- Protein containing all the essential amino acids in the correct amounts must be consumed every day; it cannot be stored in the body like fat.

- Animal proteins are the best kinds of proteins in terms of their nutritional value. Eliminating meat, milk, and eggs because of the cholesterol and fat they contain means losing the high-quality protein and other essential nutrients they provide.

- Plant proteins can provide the essential amino acids only if they are carefully chosen to balance one another.
- An all-protein diet is not healthy since it will overtax your kidneys; you need other foods as well.
- When eating high-fat foods, it is important to eat protein at the same time.

CHAPTER 4: Cutting out Carbs is Not the Answer to Weight Loss

We often associate carbohydrates (carbs) with eating sweets and breads, but carbohydrates are more than that. Carbs too, like fat, seem to be getting a bad name in nutrition. And just like fats, carbohydrates also have nutritional value. Did you know that:

- Carbohydrates (sugar and glycogen) are very important energy sources for the heart, brain, and muscles.
- It is better to get your energy from carbohydrates and fats than from protein.
- An excess of carbohydrates is made into fat in the body.
- Frequent snacks between meals actually increase weight gain more than if those same foods were eaten at wider intervals of time.
- Carbohydrates as energy sources are important to our nutrition because:
    - They save proteins for other functions in the body.
    - They provide the fuel for all our bodily functions to work including the heart, lungs, brain, and digestive systems.
    - They provide some minerals and vitamins.

All carbohydrates should be used up as fuel for the body; if they are not, they turn into fat. Obesity is a risk factor for heart disease, diabetes, cancer, and possibly other diseases.

Energy sources are both simple and complex carbohydrates. Simple carbohydrates are sucrose (sugar) and other sweeteners like corn syrup. They are called "simple" because of their chemical structure consisting of a molecule of glucose. Simple table sugar chemically contains only two glucose molecules. (Actually one of those molecules is technically fructose, which is simply a different structural arrangement of that glucose molecule.) The result of their simple chemical structure is that they are soluble (or dissolve) in water and break down quickly in the body. Complex carbohydrates contain large arrays of glucose molecules in a more complex arrangement and are not water-soluble. Complex carbohydrates are the starches, grains, and cereals that we eat.

The body, like a machine, is fed fuel by food. The foods containing simple and complex carbohydrates are the most available fuels although nearly every food contains calories (fuel). The issue often is what else each food source contains to contribute to a healthy diet.

Simple Carbohydrates: Sugars

Simple carbohydrates (sugars) usually serve purely as energy sources. The one exception is when sugars combine with amino acids (proteins) to form glycoproteins. These serve in various ways in the body such as a lubricant between membranes.[214] Any sugar that the body does not use gets converted into fat.

Americans seem to enjoy sweet foods! They consumed 129.5 pounds per capita of sweeteners in 2012, including sugar and corn syrup. This is a drop from the high in 1999 of 151.6 pounds.[215] The greatest increase in sugar consumption came in the form of soft drinks, from 3.5 gallons per person in 1909 to 22.8 gallons per person in 1971, to 51 gallons per person in 2005[216] at the cost of 14.1 billion dollars. The average consumption of soft drinks have declined since 2005 to 44.7 gallons per person according to the Huffington Post.[217] In 2011, consumption was just over 44 gallons per person, the lowest since 1987. Soft drinks have recently been linked to health problems called metabolic risks. These include higher blood pressure, higher

106

fat levels in the blood, low HDL levels, and impaired glucose metabolism.[218]

Artificial Sweeteners

There are several artificial sweeteners approved for use in the U.S. today: Aspartame ("Equal" and "NutraSweet"), acesulfame-potassium ("Sunett" and "Sweet One"), Saccharin ("Sweet'N Low" and "SugarTwin), sucralose ("Splenda"), and neotame[7]. Stevia, a natural sweetener, has been approved for limited use[8]. One sweetener, cyclamate, was banned by the FDA in 1969 although it is used in other countries[219].

Aspartame, a leading sweetener, cannot really be considered a "non-caloric" sweetener since it is broken down in the digestive tract into its components that are absorbed and metabolized. These components, aspartic acid, phenylalanine, and methanol, account for the four calories per gram of aspartame. However, since the substance is about 180 times sweeter than sugar, very little needs to be used in foods and beverages to achieve a satisfactory degree of sweetness. Diet drinks normally contain roughly 200 milligrams of the sweetener per serving. The average total consumption is about 500 milligrams per day,[220] replacing 90 grams of sugar intake and reducing calories from 360 to two. Aspartame cannot be used in cooking or baking foods since it breaks down into its components and loses its sweetening power. Aspartame cannot be used by consumers who have an inherited condition called "phenylketonurea" because of their body's inability to metabolize phenylalanine, one of the breakdown products of the sweetener. Diet-conscious consumers are aware that a can of a soft drink (12 fluid ounces) contains 150 calories or the equivalent of 10 teaspoons of sugar. They are now spending a total of 4.2 billion dollars for sugar-free soft drinks. Ironically, at the same time consumers are drinking soft drinks of any kind, they may be munching potato chips or other high calorie food. These snack foods supply more calories than would a soft drink with sugar.[23]

Artificial sweeteners are among the most controversial food additives due to allegations of adverse health effects. These allegations include dermatological problems, headaches, allergic reactions, mood swings, behavior changes, respiratory difficulties, seizures, and cancer. A very large number of studies on these substances have been carried out with conclusions ranging from "safe under all conditions" to "unsafe at any dose." Scientists are divided on the issue of artificial sweetener safety, even to the point that some researchers seem to arrive at results that confirm their own personal views. In scientific, as well as in lay publications, supporting studies are often widely referenced while the opposing results are de-emphasized or dismissed.

Artificial sweeteners add absolutely nothing to the biological value of the diet, although they cater to the "sweet tooth" of the consumer. Biologically, food is supposed to provide something of use to the body. Artificial sweeteners act more like an entertainment. Diabetics with a "sweet tooth" can continue to eat a sweet tasting food with the artificial sweetener and suffer no ill effects from the sweet taste. The replacement of sugar by artificial sweeteners in the diet may be of importance in weight reduction, in the maintenance of dental health, and in making available a greater variety of foods for diabetics, although they do not prevent overall sugar absorbtion.[221] There is some evidence that they play an opposite role in weight reduction; those using artificial sweeteners may actually be gaining weight.[222] I prefer sweeteners to come from natural substances since we may be unaware of any long-term effects from artificial substances in the body.

Complex Carbohydrates: Starches

Americans get 22% of their calories from starchy foods like bread and other baked goods, rice noodles and pastas, potatoes, vegetables, and fruits—all "complex" carbohydrates.[23] These starches are made up of simple sugars, just as proteins are made up of amino acids and fats are composed of smaller units like fatty acids and glycerin. Just as extra sugar changes to fat for energy storage, so complex carbohydrates change to fat, if not needed by the body to fuel muscle activity and provide heat so as to keep the body temperature at 98°F or 37°C. The body seems to have an unlimited capacity to store food as fat. A small amount of reserve energy is stored differently in the muscles and the liver as glycogen—a form of sugar.

Grains and Cereals. These are our major sources of fuel, and they also provide some fat and protein as well as minerals and vitamins. Cereal products include bread and other baked goods, macaroni, noodles, rice, grits, and corn meal. These products often end up for the consumer in a less nutritious form than desirable. For example, some cereals are called "whole grain." While they are made from whole grains, they often do not contain all the nutrients of the "whole" grain. Figure 10 in an earlier chapter illustrates this.

Wheat. Wheat is the most popular grain in the diet in America. However, the form of wheat we eat is less nutritious than it could be. The whole grain of wheat contains more protein than the final milled product since milling removes important nutrients. Millions of pounds of protein, along with a high percentage of the B-vitamins and iron, are removed each year through the processing of wheat alone.[223] Why are these nutrients removed? Some consumers object to the "dirty" color of flour containing bran and germ. Also white flour will not spoil as quickly as flour still containing wheat germ oil. To get more whole grain into the American diet, at least two important changes are needed:

the milling process will have to change to retain more nutrients, and consumers need to change eating habits and preferences.

Early attempts to persuade the public to use whole-grain products were unsuccessful. "Enrichment" then became the prime vehicle for getting nutrients into the diet. Since World War II the B-vitamins—thiamin, niacin, folic acid, and riboflavin—and the mineral, iron, have been added to the following products: commercially produced flour, at least 90% of standard commercial white bread, most ready-to-eat breakfast cereals, self-rising flour, corn meal, pasta such as spaghetti or ravioli, and rice. One nutrient not restored after milling is protein.

Here's a technical description of what happens during milling.[223] When wheat, corn, and rice are milled, the outer bran covering and germ portion are removed from the endosperm (the starchy part of the kernel). Although protein is found in all tissues of cereal grains, it is more concentrated in the germ (the undeveloped seed in the kernel), the scutellun (the part surrounding the germ) and the aleurone layer (the outer part of the endosperm that is removed with bran). The protein concentration increases from center to outside of the endosperm, with more protein in the aleurone and germ than in other parts of the kernel. In milling, the aleurone and germ are removed because of their objectionable color and their fat, which can become rancid. The protein in these removed fractions is not restored, although other nutrients are added back in like vitamin B_1, B_2, iron, and more recently folic acid and sometimes calcium. About 72% of the wheat kernel appears in white flour. Leftover bran and germ go mainly into livestock feed. The same consumers who insist on white flour may turn around and buy the formerly rejected portion as a health food in the form of wheat germ or bran. One way to view protein loss is that a grain of wheat contains about 14.6% protein, while white flour contains about 12.5% protein. That means approximately 2.1% of protein that could remain in white flour is lost in milling and goes to livestock and chicken feed. While this 2.1% may seem small, remember those essential amino acid charts? White bread had lesser amounts of those essential amino acids than did wheat bread as shown in Figure 9 in chapter 2.

Bread is typically made from some type of wheat flour, but its nutritional value varies greatly depending on how the flour is milled and what else has been added to the bread. Enriched bread contains various kinds of vitamins and iron, but which ones are added is not always consistent. In the United States, the FDA has mandated that folic acid (a B vitamin) be added to white bread; wheat bread, they believe, contains enough folic acid naturally. Folic acid helps prevent the occurrence of Spina Bifida (see section on vitamins later). Bread in some other countries such as in Europe is a higher protein bread because it is baked from flour with a higher extraction rate than flour in the United States.[23] The higher the extraction rate, the more whole kernel is retained in the flour. In some countries such as in Eastern Europe, even when the flour has the same essential amino acid composition as in the U.S., bakers there fortified their bread with dried yeast as a protein source. These breads have a better texture and flavor, although not as long a shelf life as American bread. Ingredients added to American bread increase its shelf life. The nutritional value of American bread could be improved by adding whey (a byproduct from cheese making), by adding Torula yeast from wood pulp processing and by adding vitamin B_6 and B_{12} and magnesium. As you can see, breads offer a wide range of nutrients and complex carbohydrates; reading the labels may be necessary to identify them specifically.

Wheat consumption may also lead to problems for some people aside from any nutrients that have or have not been added. Wheat flour contains gluten. Gluten traps the carbon dioxide formed by the fermenting yeast in the bread

111

dough causing it to rise. In some people, gluten causes changes in the lining of the small intestine resulting in malabsorption and a variety of unpleasant symptoms. This malabsorption is known as celiac disease. Once people stop eating products containing gluten, the symptoms disappear.[224] Gluten-free products are now readily available in most stores. However, some vigilance may still be needed because the substitute grains are milled at the same place as wheat and some traces of gluten remain in the next grain through the mill.

Corn. More corn is produced in the U.S. than wheat, but more wheat is consumed directly than any other cereal. About 45% of the corn crop goes to livestock feed, 42% to ethanol production, and 13% winds up for food consumption including fresh corn, cornstarch, corn sugar, dextrin (a thickener), and corn oil. [225] Corn has far less protein than wheat, and also loses protein in milling. Corn grits and corn hominy are highly refined and have lost nutritional value with both the germ and bran removed. Whole corn meal has good nutritional value, but is hard to find in grocery stores; 95% of its original kernel remains after milling. Old-fashioned, stone-ground and water-ground cornmeal also have little germ and bran removed and are better nutritional values.[23]

Rice. Rice is polished free of bran for reasons similar to the milling of wheat and corn. It has better keeping quality, freedom from rancidity, and consumer preference for white (i.e., "clean looking") rice. After World War II, the Rice Study Group considered imposing standards for lighter milling (less polishing) of rice. They decided however, that was impossible since many mills were not equipped for light milling, and because most consumers would not accept unpolished or brown rice. Wheat yields about 1.5 times as much edible food as rice. It takes 162 pounds of rough or paddy rice to yield 100 pounds of milled rice. The highest rice yields are found in brown rice or in a parboiled form.

(Parboiled rice is partially boiled, which makes the starch easier to digest and requires less cooking time.) Yields are slightly less for lightly milled or under milled rice and much lower for highly milled, polished rice. Profits in the United States are in the by-products, not milled rice. By-products include broken rice for food processing industries and for breweries and livestock food, rice polishings with their high fat content for fattening swine, and rice bran for cattle feed. Rice hulls may be used as fuel for operating the steam power plants of rice mills.

Other Cereals. Other cereal products might become popular, if consumer attitudes about "dirty" flour and rice change. Bulgur, for instance, is whole wheat that is parboiled, dried, and partially debranned. It is normally cracked to grits, which reduces cooking time and toughness. Another form of debranned whole kernel wheat food is WURLD wheat that is generally not available to consumers in the U.S.[23] Specialty breads fortified with soy or milk proteins and vitamins are available, however, at greater cost than ordinary bread.

The Effect of Too Many Carbohydrates
The purpose of carbohydrates is to produce energy. When carbohydrates (either simple or complex) are consumed in excess, the body synthesizes or changes them into fatty acids, commonly called fat. These fatty acids have only energy value, but no additional nutritional value beyond that. If you overeat, it is better to consume more animal and vegetable fat than more carbohydrates since the fat has additional nutritional value beyond its calories. The chapter on Fats explains more on this subject.

An abundance of food items high in calories, furnished by sugar, carbohydrates and/or fat, may tip the nutritional scale. If the body does not need the energy, for example, it converts the sugar or carbohydrates into fat. It takes about 4,000 calories from sugar or carbohydrates to turn into one pound of fat. These foods are easy to consume; they often are cheaper, tastier, or more convenient than other less advertised, nutritious foods. When sugars and carbohydrates come from sources like doughnuts, cookies, cream pies, and French fries, calories and fat intake skyrocket.[23]

When obesity results, some people go to the other extreme: high protein, no carbohydrate. This also imbalances the diet and is hard on the kidneys. The solution is a balanced intake of nutrients in moderation. When excess calories are consumed, they need to be "burned up" through physical work or exercise.

Some may believe that decreasing sugar consumption and increasing starch consumption may be a way to avoid gaining weight; this is based on the observation that sugar is absorbed more rapidly from the intestinal tract than starch, and if in over-supply, the sugar will be converted to fat in the body. However, in the long run, since starch (carbohydrate) foods also are converted to fat if not used as muscle energy or body heat, it is best not to over consume them as well.

CHAPTER 4 : Key Points

- Carbohydrates provide "fuel" for your body.

- Having some carbohydrates in your diet is good for you.

- You need the energy provided by carbohydrates so that your body does not have to use protein for this and overtax your kidneys.

- It's best not to overdo carbohydrates since any excess turns into fat. Eat all things in moderation!

CHAPTER 5: Your Body Needs Fiber: Your mother was right—eat your vegetables (and fruits)!

Fruits and vegetables are important parts of your diet, but are not enough in and of themselves. They have a digestible portion with nutrients, and a non-digestible part, the fiber. Did you know that:

- You need to eat a variety of fruits and vegetables for maximum benefit, not just one kind.
- Fruits and vegetables provide needed vitamins and minerals to spark processes in the body.
- Fiber provides bulk to carry the food through the intestinal tract so that nutrients can be extracted.
- Fiber carries and even speeds up the movement of fat and cholesterol through the body leaving less behind to cause problems. They carry these through the intestinal track and help keep some of it from being absorbed.
- They help to eliminate the waste products faster so that they don't overstay in the intestinal tract.
- They provide a feeling of fullness so that you stop eating.

There is good nutritional sense in eating fruits, vegetables, and grains, but not exclusively. Humans are not ruminants. Ruminants are hoofed animals that eat grass; they have an extra stomach where food can "ruminate." The human digestive system would not do well on an exclusive diet of high-bulk plants because it doesn't have that extra stomach, but it does need some bulk. You may recall that some vegetables also provide protein, but again the human body is not set up to exclusively live on vegetables that provide both protein and bulk. Those who try to do so may experience upset stomachs and diarrhea. Eating too many vegetables and having too much bulk actually seems to remove needed trace minerals from the body. Thus it is possible to have "too much of a good thing."

The "bulk" in human diets comes from fibers, the non-digestible components of fruits, vegetables, and grains. Many fibers by themselves have no food value, but in spite of that they are very important to nutrition. There are different kinds of fibers but one thing they have in common is that they all absorb water. It is important to have a variety of fibers, not just fibers from one source such as only vegetables. Together they are more effective in moving food through the intestine.

Kinds of Fibers

There are two kinds of fibers, soluble and insoluble. Soluble means they dissolve in water; they contain some nutrients that are slowly absorbed through the digestive tract. The insoluble ones do not dissolve in water; they are resistant to the digestive enzymes and essentially carry nutrients with them throughout the digestive tract. Both play roles in nutrition. Table 8 gives examples of the two kinds of fibers.

Table 8: Sources of Insoluble and Soluble Fibers in Our Diet [226]

Insoluble Fibers			Soluble Fibers	
Cellulose	Hemicellulose	Lignin	Pectin	Gums
bran	vegetables	bran	fruits	barley
whole grain	fruits	fruit skins	beets	dried beans
fruits	nuts	nuts	legumes	oat bran & oatmeal
vegetables	grains	grains	some vegetables	rye

116

Cellulose is a primary component of plants. Trees, for example, are made up of cellulose but so are many grains, and parts of fruits and vegetables. Cellulose is not digestible by humans. It is a primary carrier of food through the intestinal tract so that nutrients can be absorbed at slower rates; it carries the nutrients by absorbing water, often up to six times its weight. Cellulose also prevents the absorption of some of the cholesterol that comes from food sources. Natural forms of cellulose are preferable. The purified cellulose used in high fiber bread, for example, is limited in water absorption properties and is not the same chemically as "natural" fiber.

Hemicellulose also comes from plants and is in almost all cell walls. It is found along with cellulose in lesser amounts in grains, but in greater amounts in fruits and vegetables. It is also not digestible, but works the same way as cellulose.

Lignin is a chemical compound in plants that acts like a glue to cement cellulose and hemicelluose in the plant wall to make it somewhat rigid. Its role is the same as cellulose.

Pectin is a soluble chemical substance. It is an edible thickening agent that is often used commercially in food processing. For example, in making jelly from fruit, without pectin the fruit would end up a liquid. Pectin keeps it as a solid and hence allows for longer storage and use of the fruit. Pectin furnishes some sugar-like compounds, but they are absorbed more slowly than regular sugar. Thus it allows for longer lasting energy in the body. For example, it is better to eat an orange for your sweet tooth and for energy than to eat a cookie since the former is more slowly absorbed in the body. Pectin also helps to remove bile-acid (cholic acid) from the intestine that is the metabolized products of cholesterol. Another form of pectin, called calcium pectate, comes from leafy green vegetables. It furnishes calcium to the body. Thus eating those leafy green vegetables serves two purposes in providing us with both calcium and bulk.

Gums are soluble chemical substances in grains. They harden when exposed to air, but dissolve when in water. Gums hold nutrients together as they pass through the digestive system and allow for their slower absorption. Gums are also used in food processing to produce consistency in food ingredients. For example, gums are added to ice cream to keep the ingredients from melting too quickly.

Fiber Sources and Amounts

As you can see below, Table 9 shows the recommended daily allowances of fiber at various age groups.

Table 9: The Amount of Fiber Recommended Daily[226]

Gender, Age (years)	RDA in Grams
All children, 4-8	25
Boys, 14-18	38
Girls, 14-18	26
Men, 19-50	38
Women, 19-50	25
Men, over 50	30
Women, over 50	21

It is estimated that Americans get far less fiber than the recommended amount in their daily diets, perhaps less than half of what they need.[227] Table 11 points out various sources of fiber and how much a typical serving provides. You can see how you need to eat several fiber-rich foods to meet your daily requirement.

The water-holding capacity and absorptive properties vary with the fruit and vegetable sources of fiber. Fiber from fruits and vegetables is more fermentable and digestible than "mature" fiber from grains such as bran. Carrot, orange, and apple fibers hold a lot of water relative to wheat bran, although coarse bran absorbs some six times its weight in water and fine bran, three times. Remember that a variety of fibers are needed because of their different characteristics.

Fiber as a Fat-Fighter and Health Benefit

Fiber functions effectively as a fat-fighter since it expands inside the stomach, filling and satisfying without calories. When adequate quantities of fiber from fruits, vegetables, and cereals are consumed, there is less inclination to consume empty-calorie foods high in fat and sugar.

Table 10: Sources of Fiber. In grams/100 grams[227]

Food	Amount of Fiber	Food	Amount of Fiber
Grains			
Barley, pearled	3.8	Rice, raw (brown)	5.5
Cornmeal, whole grain	11	Rice, raw (white)	1-2.8
De-germed wheat	5.2	Rice, raw (wild)	5.2
Oat bran, raw	6.6	Wheat bran	15
Vegetables			
Broccoli, raw	7.7	Corn, sweet, cooked	3.7
Brussels sprouts, cooked	2.6	Edible pod peas, raw	2.6
Cabbage (white), raw	2.4	Potatoes, white, baked, w/ skin	5.5
Carrots	3.2	Sweet potato, cooked	3
Cauliflower, raw	2.4	Tomatoes, raw	1.3
Fruits			
Apples (w/ skin)	2.8	Pears (raw)	2.6
Apricots (dried)	7.8	Prunes (dried)	7.2
Bananas	1.8	Prunes (stewed)	6.6
Figs (dried)	9.3	Raisins	5.3
Bread			
Bagel	2.1	Pita bread (whole wheat)	4.7
Bran bread	8.5	White bread	1.9
Pita bread (white)	1.6	Whole wheat bread	2.0
Cereals			
Bran cereal	35.3	Granola bar	6.2
Bran flakes	18.8	Oatmeal	10.6
Cornflakes	2	Wheat flakes	9
Nuts			
Almonds, oil-roasted	11.2	Peanuts, dry-roasted	8
Coconut, raw	9	Pistachios	10.8
Hazelnuts, oil-roasted	6.4	Cashews	9.3
Beans			
Baked beans (vegetarian)	7.7	Chickpeas, canned	5.4
Black beans, cooked	10.8	Lima beans, cooked	7.2
Others			
Corn chips, toasted	4.4	Tofu	1.2

Fiber also provides important specific health benefits, especially in digestion. For example, bulk-containing foods

119

tend to lower blood cholesterol levels. Cholesterol is eventually converted into bile acids that help eliminate cholesterol from the body; fiber helps in that elimination process. Substances called saponins in foods such as beets, asparagus, soybeans, eggplant, pineapple, spinach, yams, and oats probably also have a cholesterol-lowering effect.[228,229]

Fibers contain and carry some of the important minerals, such as calcium and magnesium. They also contain and carry some important trace minerals such as silicon, iron, and zinc. However, eating too much fiber seems to eliminate some of these vital minerals from the body.

Fiber permits enzymes to digest food more slowly in the intestinal tract, resulting in a slower release of sugar.[230] This is effective in diabetes management. Studies suggest that high fiber consumption counteracts the effect of excess salt on hypertension.[231] By virtue of its relative indigestibility, fiber is non-fattening.

Fiber seems to provide a way for cholesterol to ride through the body and not be turned into the "bad stuff." It is interesting that the study[12] on cholesterol absorption in the body was carried out on patients on a liquid diet without fiber. In that study, 34-63% of the cholesterol was absorbed. It is highly likely that had the diet contained fiber, this figure would be far less. Fiber seems to protect against high cholesterol levels, as well as reduce the excretion of bile acids and prevent the rapid absorption of sugar.[232]

Fiber and the Body's Waste Products
Increased fiber leads to increased waste output, including larger stools. It also shortens digestive transit time enabling people to pass their waste daily, and it increases softness of chime (the medical term for stools) due to increased moisture content. When food stays longer in the intestinal tract, the results may be constipation and/or more time for nasty bacteria like Escherichia (E) coli to grow to

excess and create problems. Fiber helps keep things moving, so to speak.

No section on fiber would be complete without talking about a side product, called "fermentation hydrogen" in biochemical terms or "flatulence" in the medical terminology or … well I won't go into the common vernacular. It is the increased amount of gas accumulated in the digestive tract. As food moves through the digestive tract, some food ferments more than others. Typically these foods are high in fiber, such as beans and cabbage, although there are other foods such as milk products that can cause this as well. More fermentation means more flatulence. Thus it is important to keep food moving throughout the body so that there is less opportunity for that fermentation. For some people this means eating more fiber, but for others, it means eating less fiber. When you are alone for a day or more, you may wish to experiment as to which category you're in.

CHAPTER 5 : Key Points

- Foods with fibers provide needed vitamins and minerals and help carry food throughout our bodies.
- Make sure you eat a variety of grains, fruits and vegetables daily, not one exclusively.
- Don't overdo on fibers (you're not a cow), because fibers can wash out needed minerals.
- One cannot exist on fiber alone, so include the other foods as well.

CHAPTER 6: A Multivitamin May do More Harm than Good: The minerals, vitamins and antioxidants you need (or don't)

Vitamins, minerals, and antioxidants are already in your diet if you eat the sources of food we suggested in the previous chapters. Without these, your health is likely to suffer. Did you know that:

- Minerals help regulate the blood flow in the body—keeping it flowing when it should, and clotting when necessary.
- Minerals and vitamins help regulate the heartbeat.
- Minerals and vitamins help build healthy bones.
- Minerals and vitamins prevent a whole host of diseases.
- Antioxidants prevent the oxidation of polyunsaturated fats; that is they keep the fats from being used in a negative way by the body.
- It's better to get your vitamins and minerals through your diet than through pills because the pills likely contain more than you need and the body, in some cases, cannot handle the excess well.

The best sources of vitamins and minerals come from eggs, meat, milk products, vegetables, fruits, nuts, and grains.[233] No additional supplements are needed if you include these foods in your diet.

Minerals

Minerals are needed in our bodies because:

- They provide structure to the bones; bones are made up of calcium and phosphate, magnesium, and protein and a number of trace minerals.[234]

- They carry out metabolic processes, the processes required for us to live. For example, sodium, calcium, magnesium, and potassium are required to stimulate the heartbeat and carry nerve impulses.[233]

- They are a necessary component of enzymes that carry on the life process. For example, iron is needed in the red blood cells to carry oxygen. Enzymes act as catalysts or the means to get a particular biochemical process started. It's like a spark to start a fire. Enzyme systems include a vitamin, a mineral, and a protein.

Table 11 provides a summary of the essential minerals—what they do, their sources, and the Recommended Daily Allowance (RDA).[214]

Some minerals are considered "essential" while others are not. An essential element is one whose deficiency produces repeated structural and physiological abnormalities; when that mineral is added back in the diet, that abnormality is reversed.[235] Then there are macro-minerals and micro-minerals; these are related to the amounts the body needs. If the amount of the mineral needed is in milligrams (mg), it is called a macro-mineral whereas those elements present in microgram (mcg) quantities are designated as trace minerals or microminerals. (As a point of reference, one ounce equals approximately 28.5 grams or 28,349 milligrams and 1000 mcg=1 mg.)

Calcium, magnesium, sodium, and potassium are called the macroelements because they are needed in larger quantities than the microminerals, such as copper, zinc, etc. The role of the so-called microminerals, or trace elements, is newer in the nutrition field. We now know that they are very important to the life process because they are a necessary component of enzymes, which carry out the metabolic process in living cells. Vitamins must be combined with a mineral (also called a metal) and protein to serve as an enzyme to become involved in the thousands of chemical reactions that make life possible. On the other hand, if a little is good, a lot is not always better—some of the micronutrients such as selenium are highly toxic in larger doses. First we'll discuss the macro-minerals. With each one in the text, we'll also include its scientific abbreviation in parentheses after its name.

Table 11. Summary of Essential Minerals[214]

Macrominerals			
Mineral	*Function*	*Sources*	*RDA*
Calcium	Essential for developing and maintaining healthy bones and teeth. Assists in blood clotting, muscle contraction, nerve transmission. Reduces risk of osteoporosis.	Dairy products, green leafy vegetables (except spinach), canned fish, tofu.	No RDAs have been set for calcium. These values are considered to be "Adequate Intakes." 19–50 years old: 1000 mg 51+ years old: 1,200 mg
Phosphorus	Works with calcium to	Dairy products,	19+ years old:

	develop and maintain strong bones and teeth. Enhances use of other nutrients. Essential for energy metabolism, DNA structure, and cell membranes.	meats, poultry, fish, eggs, whole grains, nuts and seeds, processed foods.	700 mg
Magnesium	Activates nearly 100 enzymes and helps nerves and muscles function.	Green vegetables, legumes, cereal, fish, and whole bran.	19+ years old *Women: 320 mg* *Men: 420 mg*
Sodium	Necessary for maintaining fluid balance. Transports nutrients across cell membranes.	Table salt, milk, processed meats (luncheon meats, ham, bacon), snack chips, crackers.	There is no RDA for sodium.

Potassium	Maintaining fluid balance.	Spinach, Brussels sprouts, bananas, potatoes, tomatoes, orange juice, and cantaloupe.	No RDA has been established for potassium. This value is considered to be a minimum daily requirement 2000 mg.
Chloride	Necessary for maintaining normal acidity in the stomach. Helps carry carbon dioxide to the lungs.	Table salt.	No RDA has been established for chloride, but the value below is considered to be the minimum daily requirement 750 mg.
Iron	Needed for red blood cell formation and function.	Liver, meats, green leafy vegetables, enriched breads and cereals.	19+ years old: 8 mg 19–50 years old: 18 mg 51+ years old: 8 mg
Trace Minerals or Microminerals			

Mineral	Function	Sources	RDA
Zinc	Essential part of more than 100 enzymes involved in digestion, metabolism, reproduction and normal wound healing.	Meat, liver, poultry, fish, oysters, other seafood, whole grains, eggs.	19+ years old Men: 11 mg Women: 8 mg
Iodine	Helps regulate growth, development, and metabolism. Necessary for normal thyroid function.	Iodized salt, saltwater fish, dairy products, white bread.	19+ years old: 150 mcg
Selenium	Necessary for normal growth, development, use of iodine in thyroid function.	Whole grains, fish, seafood, liver, meats, eggs.	55 mcg
Copper	Involved in iron metabolism, nervous system	Liver, seafood, nuts, seeds.	19+ years old: 900 mcg

	function, bone health, synthesis of proteins and pigmentation of skin, hair, eyes.		
Manganese	Necessary for normal development of skeletal and connective tissues. Involved in carbohydrate metabolism	Whole grains, cereals.	No RDAs have been set for manganese. These values are considered to be "Adequate Intakes." <u>19+ years old</u> *Men: 2.3 mg - Women: 1.8 mg*
Fluoride	Dental health and incorporation into bones and teeth.	Most plants and animals, fluoride-fortified toothpaste, some water supplies.	No RDAs have been set for fluoride. These values are considered to be "Adequate Intakes." <u>19+ years old</u> *Men: 4.0 mg - Women: 3.0 mg*

Chromium	Needed for normal glucose metabolism	Egg yolks, whole grains, pork.	No RDAs have been set for chromium. These values are considered to be "Adequate Intakes." <u>19–50 years old</u> *Men: 35 mcg - Women: 25 mcg* <u>51+ years old</u> *Men: 30 mcg - Women: 20 mcg*
Molybdenum	Needed for metabolism of DNA and RNA.	Milk, beans, breads, cereals.	19+ years old: 45 mcg

From *The Merck Manual of Medical Information – Second Home Edition*, p. 902-903, edited by Mark H. Beers. Copyright 2013 by Merck & Co., Inc., Whitehouse Station, NJ. Availableat:http://www.merck.com/mmhe/sec12/ch154/ch154a.html?qt=vitamins&alt=sh . Accessed (2013).

Calcium (Ca)

Calcium is an essential element required for bone structure, for the use of muscles, for blood clotting and for several life processes, particularly for the normal contraction of the heart.[235] The daily requirement of calcium is best met by drinking milk and eating milk products like cheese and green leafy vegetables. Imitation cheese, made from soybean protein and used in products such as pizzas, does not contain calcium either in spite of its name. For those who don't like milk or are lactose intolerant, there are other natural sources of calcium. Table 12 lists sources of calcium. Calcium tablets are not good substitutes for foods that contain calcium if they contain calcium carbonate or calcium oxide because these are poorly absorbed from the intestines.

Table 12: Sources of Calcium[234]

Calcium Rich Foods	Amount for 1 Serving (3-4 servings/day recommended)
Milk	1 cup+ or 250mL
Cheese (Cheddar, Edam, Gouda)	1 1/4" or 3 cm cube
Cheese – Mozzarella	1 1/4" or 3 cm cube
Yogurt	3/4 cup or 185 mL
Green leafy vegetables	1/2 cup or 125 mL
Canned fish (with bones)	1/2 can or 105 g
Tofu (with calcium sulfate)	3 oz or 84 g

Calcium is necessary to make muscles work. All muscles, including the heart and the blood vessels, need calcium to make them expand and contract. The heart does not store extra calcium like the bones do, so that calcium in our daily diets is essential. The heart is profoundly affected when calcium is deficient in the diet.[235] Popular drugs, such as beta blockers, attempt to regulate the flow of calcium to heart cells.

Sodium (Na) and Potassium (K)
Sodium and potassium are discussed together because they work in tandem. They are essential constituents of three body fluids: cell plasma (cytoplasm), lymph, and

blood. Here's how these body fluids work together: The cell cytoplasm is a liquid inside the cell (the cytosol) surrounded by the plasma membrane. Lymph, also a liquid, is outside of the cells and provides the environment that "bathes" the cells. Blood brings the nutrients to the cells. Sodium and potassium maintain the balance between the three liquids in the body and protect the cell so that no one liquid overpowers the other.[236] Fruits and vegetables are rich sources of potassium. Potassium rich foods such as banana and cantaloupe are usually low in sodium. A recommended daily allowance has not been established for potassium although 2000 mg is thought to be a minimum daily requirement. Table 13 presents the potassium amounts in a variety of foods.

Table 13. Food Sources and Amounts of Potassium (K)[237]

Foods	Serving	K (mg)	Foods	Serving	K (mg)
Apple	1 med.	143	Kidney beans, canned	8 oz.	343
Apricot, fresh	1 med.	107	Lettuce, iceberg	3.5 oz.	175
Banana	1 med.	555	Lettuce, romaine	3.5 oz.	264
Dates, dried	1 ea.	65	Onion	1 med.	157
Grapes, green seedless	1 cup	220	Peas, fresh cooked	8 oz.	98
Orange Juice, fresh	8 oz.	250	Potato, baked w/ skin	1 med.	503
Papaya	1 large	936	Pumpkin, canned	4 oz.	180
Peach	1 med.	234	Spinach, steamed	8 oz.	167
Pineapple, fresh	1 cup	204	Sweet Potato	1 sm.	300
Prune Juice	8 oz.	284	Tomato	1 med.	366
Raisins	4 oz.	305	Ice Cream	8 oz.	105
Strawberries, fresh	1 cup	244	Milk, skim	8 oz.	178
Asparagus, cooked	1 spear	29	Yogurt, low fat	8 oz.	178
Artichoke	1 sm.	300	Bread, wheat	1 slice	59
Foods	Serving	K (mg)	Foods	Serving	K (mg)
Broccoli	1 cup	401	Brazil nuts	4 oz.	540
Cabbage, cooked	1 cup	277	Egg	1 med.	65
Celery, raw	1 lg stalk	171	Hamburger	4 oz.	383
Corn, on cob	1 med.	165	Peanuts, roasted w/skin	4 oz.	404
Green Beans	8 oz.	95	Peanut butter, natural	1 tbsp.	94
Green Pepper	1 lg.	213	Rice, brown	1 cup	105
Rice, white	1 cup	42	Salmon, canned	4 oz.	409

The sodium content of natural and processed foods is most likely sufficient to provide for your sodium demand. If not, you can always add salt to your food. Too much salt, however, can have detrimental effects including elevated blood pressure, in some people.

Magnesium (Mg)

Magnesium has been shown to be essential in more than 100 enzyme systems; it acts like a spark to start life in the body. Just a few of the ways magnesium is important to our bodies are included here. Calcium and magnesium are both part of bone structure. Magnesium is needed as a cofactor for the enzymes that convert the essential fatty acids into a form that helps regulate blood flow.[238,239] Magnesium is needed for our muscles to contract properly. Magnesium also helps our heart to work. It's been suggested the lack of magnesium in the diet may be a cause of the sudden deaths from heart attacks of young and middle-aged men in the prime of life as well as the development of heart disease throughout the population.[240] Magnesium deficiency has been implicated in a host of diseases including heart disease (with increased risk of blood clots and heart attacks), cancer, immune function, Alzheimer's disease, osteoporosis, stroke, and neurological diseases.[235]

Table 14 shows several sources of magnesium. Sea salt used in the U.S., Canada, and Western Europe contains magnesium, calcium, and potassium as well as sodium. This salt is available in grocery stores and to commercial livestock producers resulting in magnesium being present in meat.

Table 14. Sources of Magnesium[241]

Magnesium Sources
Hard water
Sea salt
Green leafy vegetables
Nuts
Cereals, such as oat, wheat and corn

Magnesium intake has been progressively decreasing in industrialized countries over the past century, and this decrease has been related to the increase in cardiovascular disease and hypertension.[240] Several studies have also suggested that magnesium intake is inadequate in the U.S. population.[238,239] The group most likely to have deficient magnesium would be those taking diuretics commonly prescribed for hypertension and other cardiovascular disorders.[242] This medication increases the urine flow and pulls magnesium out of the body. Other groups at risk would be chronic alcoholics, those in a state of severe malnutrition, and those with bowel diseases. Magnesium depletion may cause severe muscle spasms, coma, and death.

Epidemiologists have compared the lower death rates from coronary heart disease in Japan, China, India, Italy, and Greece to higher death rates from coronary heart disease in the U.S. and Northern Europe. They speculate that differences in the diet, specifically more saturated fats and higher cholesterol intake, account for their observations. I think another explanation may have relevance—the composition of the salt used in all those countries may have contributed to the differences in death rates. The table salt uscd in Japan, India, Italy, and Greece is obtained by evaporating ocean water and therefore contains calcium, magnesium, and potassium in addition to sodium. The Japanese consume 10 grams of ocean salt per day. That salt would supply approximately 1500 milligrams of magnesium per day or almost twice as much as the US National Research Council recommended requirement. The table salt available in the U.S. and Northern Europe is obtained from salt mines and loses its magnesium, calcium, and potassium as a result of its processing. Americans consume approximately 5 grams of U.S. table salt per day; their salt lacks those essential minerals. Is the lower rate of heart disease in Japan, China, India, Italy, and Greece due to a higher magnesium intake? Is their higher rate of death from hypertension and cerebral strokes due to a higher sodium intake? We can only speculate.

The high percentage of fat and sugar in the American diet requires a greater need for magnesium-rich foods to be consumed along with the fat and sugars since magnesium aids in their digestion and serves as a means of lowering cholesterol.[194] Diets high in fat, salt, phosphate, calcium, and vitamin D increase magnesium requirements and intensify any magnesium deficiency. The magnesium intake in Western European countries and in the U.S. averages 329 milligrams per day. There is disagreement as to whether this is an adequate amount. Studies in which people were fed fruits, vegetables, and grains rich in magnesium (605-1140 milligrams per day) showed decreased incidence of heart disease.[250] In animal studies, magnesium seems to be protective against heart damage. With enough magnesium in the diet, trans fat is not as harmful.[4,185] Breastfeeding women would be well-advised to increase their dietary magnesium intake.

Hard water contains a high concentration of minerals, specifically calcium and magnesium. However, most water sources are not hard; almost all major cities get their water from nearby rivers, which do not have minerals in high quantities, or soften the water for residents and thereby reduce magnesium concentrations.[243] Drinking "hard" water with higher concentrations of magnesium seems to protect against cardiovascular disease, including stroke and hypertension.[244] The muscle cells in the heart are depleted of magnesium within a few minutes after a heart attack.[245] It may be judicious to add magnesium, calcium, sodium, and potassium to the glucose used in intravenous solutions to restore these minerals to the blood in patients in intensive care facilities. These minerals could be used in the same percentage found in blood to restore them more rapidly to the recuperating cardiac cells. Research in Europe has found this to be helpful, but in the U.S. this has not yet been demonstrated.

The need for magnesium in cases of extreme thirst (dehydration) was evident to me in a chance conversation with General Schweigart who was in charge of nutrition in the German army during World War II. You may recall that General Rommel was named the "desert fox" by the British because of his success in fighting the British in Northern Africa. The German tank drivers were fainting in their tanks from extreme heat and dehydration in spite of extra salt pills. General Schweigart ordered that a pint of milk (which naturally contains magnesium) be added to their daily ration. I've often since wondered whether General Rommel's success in eluding the British was because the German tank drivers had magnesium and did not faint while the British tank drivers fainted in their tanks. The magnesium in that milk may have been responsible for General Rommel's success on the battlefield.

Trace Minerals

Copper, zinc, manganese, selenium, chromium, cobalt, iodine, molybdenum, and fluoride have been designated essential trace minerals.[246] Nickel, vanadium, and silicon are currently under study to determine whether they are also essential trace minerals. Remember if an essential mineral is missing, structural and physiological abnormalities of the human body occur, but those changes can be reversed by adding that element back into the diet.

Apart from these minerals, there are four nonessential trace minerals: cadmium, arsenic, mercury, and lead, present in our environment that may accumulate in one's body upon aging and exposure to them. Too much of any one of these four nonessential trace minerals leads to health problems.

Animal food products may contribute more trace minerals to the diet than cereals or legumes. Beef cattle kept on the grassland of the western U.S. have access to licking blocks of trace minerals such as copper, zinc, manganese, iron, etc., which deposit in their muscle tissue. Dairy cattle also have access to blocks of trace minerals, and swine and poultry rations contain trace minerals. As previously described, the milling process of cereals such as corn and wheat for human consumption further reduces trace minerals compared to animal food products. How important this is to the synthesis of the enzymes that require trace minerals in their chemical makeup for human nutrition is seldom considered in diet recommendations. Here's a bit more information on some trace minerals.

Copper (Cu). Some enzymes need copper, but not much of it.[247-249] Probably 1 mg/day is adequate; however, about one third of American diets contain less than this.[248] Vegetables, spices, and fruits such as bananas and apples are rich in copper. Copper deficiencies and copper excesses have been linked to heart disease although the exact relationship is unknown.[249]

Chromium (Cr). Chromium appears to be an essential trace element in humans.[250] The chromium requirement has been estimated to be around 70 micrograms per day. Low-income groups have a lower (by 25%) intake of chromium.[251] People in sedentary occupations consume approximately 70-90 micrograms per day of chromium. Even when you eat food with chromium in it, only 70-80% of it is used. Vegetables such as spinach leaves, cabbage, carrots, onion, potato, beans, celery stalks, chilies, green pepper, and black pepper are rich sources of chromium. Apples, bananas, cherries, guava, and ripe tomatoes also contain traces of chromium. Chromium not in food is absorbed only at the 1-2% level[252] so taking it by tablet is relatively ineffective. Chromium may be an important factor in the development of heart disease and diabetes.[253] Epidemiological studies show that chromium in drinking water or in the diet relates inversely to the incidence of hypertension, stroke, or coronary heart disease. Chromium may even be protective, but there are contradictory results.

Selenium (Se). Selenium is a relatively new addition to our knowledge of essential trace minerals for men and women.[254] The first descriptions of deficiency symptoms in humans were in the 1970s.[255] Food is the major source of selenium intake. Traces appear in fish, meat, and vegetables. Studies seem to show that those with low selenium levels may have more heart disease and strokes because selenium may function as an antioxidant.[256] The recommended daily intake is 50-100 micrograms per day.[257]

Minerals in Tablet Form

Many of the minerals, both macro and trace, are available in pill form. However, if you have a balanced diet, it is unnecessary to take any minerals in these forms. Minerals in our diet are likely to be in the right amounts. Minerals in pill form often contain too much of the actual mineral and can sometimes cause problems. Furthermore, they are not absorbed in the same way as the minerals in food sources, thus leading to inappropriate amounts as well.

Vitamins

Vitamins are needed in our bodies because:[257]

- They are part of an enzyme system, along with minerals and proteins.
- They help carry out metabolic processes.
- Specific vitamins help prevent specific birth defects and specific diseases.

There are essentially two kinds of vitamins: fat-soluble and water-soluble. The fat-soluble vitamins are stored in the liver and in body fat deposits and thus remain in the body for a relatively long period of time. Water-soluble vitamins are present in the body for only short periods of time. This has implications for the amounts needed daily. Table 16 identifies various vitamins, recommended amounts and food sources, as well as their functions and how a vitamin deficiency may manifest itself.

You can have too little of a vitamin, the effects of which are shown in the "deficiency" column of Table 15. For example, a lack of vitamin A leads to blindness in babies. This was shown tragically in India many years ago when skim milk powder not fortified with vitamin A was fed to babies who then went blind.[258] You can also overdo on some vitamins. For example, too much vitamin A causes severe headaches. Too much vitamin K could lead to blood clots.[145] Too much vitamin D causes calcium to deposit in the coronary arteries leading to atherosclerosis.[79] Eating foods that naturally furnish these vitamins will likely lead to correct amounts in your body.

Table 15: Vitamins[214]

Fat-Soluble Vitamins	RDA	Sources	Functions	Deficiency Symptoms
A (carotene)	5000 IU/day	Yellow or orange fruits and vegetables, green leafy vegetables, fortified oatmeal, liver, fortified dairy products	Maintenance of skin, hair, and mucous membranes. Vision in dim light. Bone growth. Immunity. Fetal development.	Night blindness, dry and scaly skin, frequent fatigue. If severe, corneal lesions, blindness.
D	400 IU/day	Fortified milk, sunlight, fish, eggs butter, fortified margarine	Aids in bone and tooth formation. Helps maintain heart actions and nervous system.	In children: rickets and other bone deformities. In adults: calcium loss from bones.
E	30 IU/day	Fortified and multi-grain cereals, nuts, wheat germ, vegetable oils, green leafy vegetables.	Protects blood cells, body tissue and essential fatty acids from harmful destruction in the body.	Muscular wasting, nerve damage, anemia, reproductive failure.
K	N/A	Green leafy vegetables, fruit, dairy and grain products	Essential for blood clotting functions; adds calcium to bones.	Bleeding disorders in infants and those on blood-thinning medications.
Co-Enzyme Q	N/A	A fat-soluble vitamin that can be made in the body or purchased.	Involved in converting Acetyl CoA to energy	Low in the blood of heart patients.
Water-Soluble	**RDA**	**Sources**	**Functions**	**Deficiency Symptoms**
B_1 (thiamin)	1.5 mg/day	Fortified cereals and other products, meats, brown rice, pasta, whole grains, liver, eggs	Helps body release energy from carbohydrates during metabolism. Growth and muscle tone.	Heart irregularity, fatigue, nerve disorders, mental confusion, Beriberi
Niacin	20 mg/day	Meat, poultry, fish, fortified cereals, bread and rice, peanuts, potatoes, dairy products, eggs	Involved in carbohydrate, protein, and fat metabolism	Skin disorders, diarrhea, indigestion, general fatigue, Pellagra
B_6 (pyridoxine)	2 mg/day	Fish, poultry, lean meats, bananas, prunes, dried beans, whole grains, avocados, eggs	Helps build body tissue and aids in metabolism of protein. Needed to generate glucose from amino acids	Convulsions, dermatitis, muscular weakness, skin cracks, anemia, mental depression
B_{12} (cobalamin)	6 mcg/day	Meats, milk products, seafood, eggs	Aids nervous system functioning, cell development, and protein and fat metabolism	Anemia, nervousness, fatigue, and, in some cases, neuritis and brain degeneration
Folate (folic acid)	0.4 mg/day	Green leafy vegetables, organ meats, dry peas, beans, lentils, fortified flour and cereals, eggs	Aids in genetic material development and is also involved in red blood cell production.	Gastrointestinal disorders, anemia, cracks on lips, spina bifida, homocystinemia
Pantothenic Acid	10 mg/day	Lean meats, whole grains, legumes, eggs, vegetables, fruits.	Helps in the release of energy from fats and carbohydrates.	Fatigue, vomiting, stomach stress, infections, muscle cramps
B_2 (riboflavin)	1.7 mg/day	Whole grains, green leafy vegetables, organ meats, milk and eggs. Added to breakfast cereal and flour in U.S.	Helps body release energy from protein, fat and carbohydrates during metabolism	Cracks in corners of mouth, skin rash, anemia
Biotin	0.3 mg/day	Cereal/grain products, yeast, legumes, liver eggs	Involved in metabolism of protein, fats and carbohydrates.	Nausea, vomiting, depression, hair loss, dry, scaly skin (dermatitis)
C (ascorbic acid)	60 mg/day	Citrus fruits, berries, and vegetables, especially peppers, fortified fruit juices and other beverages.	Essential for structure of bones, cartilage, muscle and blood vessels. Helps maintain capillaries and gums, aids in iron absorption.	Swollen or bleeding gums, slow wound healing, fatigue/depression, poor digestion, scurvy

The B Vitamins

There are a number of B vitamins, each one with its specific role as part of the enzyme systems in the body. Enzyme systems also include a mineral and a protein. Although there is a B_{12} vitamin, actually there aren't twelve B vitamins. Several substances along the way were named as B vitamins but did not pan out to be real vitamins in the long run. They were assigned a number in the discovery process and that number was not used again. Some B vitamins also were named, such as riboflavin.

The necessary roles of thiamin, riboflavin, and niacin, were recognized in the 1940s and '50s in the quest for essential nutrients and were added to flour; this addition was widely accepted. Vitamins such as folic acid, pyridoxine (B_6), cyanocobalamin (B_{12}) and coenzyme Q were discovered in the late 1950s and '60s and except for folic acid, have not yet been added to flour. Why these have been or should be added to flour is explained below.

Folic acid was added to flour in the 1990s in order to prevent spina bifida, a neural tube defect (a disorder involving incomplete development of the brain, spinal cord and/or their protective covering) caused by the failure of the fetal spine to close properly during the first month of pregnancy.[259] Although the spinal opening can be surgically repaired shortly after birth, the nerve damage is permanent, resulting in varying degrees of paralysis of the lower limbs. In addition to physical mobility, most individuals have some form of learning disability. There is no cure for spina bifida because the nerve tissue cannot be replaced or repaired. The addition of 0.4 milligrams folic acid per day to the diet of women of childbearing age significantly reduces the incidence of spina bifida.

Vitamins B_6 and B_{12} and folate help metabolize one of the essential amino acids, methionine. A compound named homocysteine occurs in small amounts naturally

142

during this process of metabolism. However, when these vitamins[260] are not present, the methionine is not used or metabolized properly and homocysteine is produced in greater amounts.[261] Vitamin B_6 makes sure that there is not too much homocysteine in your blood—if you don't have enough vitamin B_6, you end up with too much homocysteine. Too much homocysteine is believed to correlate with a high incidence of cardiovascular disease. An excess amount of homocysteine has been found in the blood of patients with heart disease and now is found in teenagers.[262] Elevated blood levels of homocysteine have been linked to increased risk of premature coronary artery disease, stroke, and thromboembolism (venous blood clots), even among people who have normal cholesterol levels.[263,264] However, a recent study showed that a supplement of 2.5mg of folic acid, 50mg vitamin B_6. and 1mg of vitamin B_{12} a day did not reduce the risk of major cardiovascular events in patients with vascular events.[265] This study was on those already with heart disease; perhaps the dosages were too high and perhaps it was too late for them. In preventing heart disease, these vitamins may have more of an impact.

In order to minimize homocysteine levels, the solution could be as simple as fortifying flour with vitamins B_6 and B_{12}. To lower the homocysteine levels of teenagers, consider what changing the ingredients of a popular food, pizza, could do. Currently, the crust is made with flour not fortified with B_6 or B_{12}. Because of fierce price competition, a soybean simulated cheese product may replace actual cheese in some pizzas because it is less expensive. Cheese, a complete protein, does contain some B_6 and B_{12}, while the soybean product is devoid of them and is an incomplete protein. With real cheese and the additions of those B vitamins, pizza could contribute much more to the nutrition of teenagers and others.

Vitamin D

Vitamin D is essential to help build our bones by helping calcium to deposit itself in our bones. However, with too much vitamin D and not enough calcium in the diet, bones get robbed of calcium, which ends up being deposited in the arteries and can lead to heart disease.[266,267] The catch with vitamin D is how much is enough and how do you avoid getting too much.

True vitamins have to come from your food; your body cannot make a vitamin. Thus, vitamin D is not a true vitamin since you can make some of it yourself by being in sunlight. Furthermore, your body stores vitamin D in your liver. So people with light skin who are outside in the summer months are likely to have enough vitamin D to last for the entire year. The amount of daily sun exposure required to get a year's worth of vitamin D is currently unknown. Exposure to the sun for 30 minutes per day may meet this requirement. Those exposed for up to eight hours did not increase this level, although they may be more at risk for skin cancer. People with dark skins may filter out more sunlight so they may need longer exposure (up to six times as much) to meet their Vitamin D requirements.[268] These times may vary, of course, with the time of day, latitude, and the season. Those who are rarely in sunlight, like the elderly, need to make sure they have adequate vitamin D through their diets or a supplement. Dietary recommendations, therefore, should be applied only to those who receive inadequate summer sun exposure.

In the U.S., to ensure that the entire population receives an adequate dietary supply of vitamin D, certain foods are fortified. These are milk, margarine, and some breakfast cereals.[269] Thus, even those people receiving adequate sunlight exposure often receive an additional dose of vitamin D in the diet. In addition, because many people are concerned with their diets, a significant portion of the American population is also increasing their normal dietary intake with vitamin supplements, sometimes in megadoses, including vitamin D.[269] This dietary supplementation and food fortification occurs despite ample evidence that an excessive intake of vitamin D can produce harmful effects, including actually removing calcium from the bones.[270]

The exact human requirement for vitamin D is not known. The DRI was recently updated to 600 IU (International Units) for most adults and 800 IU for adults over 70 years. We know that 250 IU per day prevents rickets and ensures adequate calcium absorption and bone mineralization. Rickets, by the way, is a condition in which bones are deformed; people with rickets may look very bow-legged. Most vitamin D tablets contain 400 IU. A quart of milk (four 8-ounce glasses of milk) is fortified with 400 IU.

Because infants grow so rapidly, they are particularly susceptible to diet deficiencies. Breast milk contains very little vitamin D (perhaps up to 200 IUs per quart), unless the mothers have a higher intake of Vitamin D, suggesting that infants do require additional vitamin D for their growth. Studies of infant growth substantiate this.[271,272] Sunlight may provide enough of the missing vitamin D without additional supplements.

In 1919, the discovery that vitamin D in cod liver oil prevented rickets resulted in increasing amounts of vitamin D into the American diet. Taking cod liver oil really was a good (and often necessary) thing back then! Luckily it is no longer needed. From 1923 to 1930, imports of fish liver oil increased from 531,015 gallons to 2,894,967 gallons.[273] After 1930, milk began to be irradiated with ultraviolet light. This process also produced vitamin D and people no longer needed that cod liver oil, a relief to many since it did not taste good. A patent restricted the irradiation process to milk so that milk was fortified with vitamin D, but other foods were not. However in 1947, a host of things happened leading to the abandonment of irradiation of milk and thus a change in how many people got vitamin D. First, the

Steenbock patent based on the ultraviolet exposure of milk items[274] and its vitamin D fortification was declared invalid by the Supreme Court, allowing any manufacturer who wanted to irradiate any food to do so. Second, the irradiation of the food products themselves could not be controlled well and required frequent checks. Third, chemically synthesized vitamin D was now available. Because of the simplicity of use, other foods as well as milk were fortified with the synthetic vitamin. The manufacture of synthetic vitamin D, which is inexpensive to make, increased from 35 pounds in 1948 to 14,000 pounds today.[275] Simply looking at food labels shows that vitamin D is added to baked goods, breakfast cereals, pasta, and rice dishes, fats and oils, milk and milk products, sauces, nonalcoholic beverages, and baby formulas.[276] Vitamin D was added to orange juice in April of 2005. Vitamin D-fortified breakfast cereals, milk, and infant formulas contain the highest amounts.

It is not difficult to consume well over the recommended 600 IU of vitamin D per day.[276,277] A serving of highly fortified cereal with milk for breakfast, 8 ounces of rockfish with a glass of milk for lunch, and chicken soup, plus a 4-ounce serving of meat, and a vanilla pudding dessert at dinner would supply over 2280 IU of vitamin D.[278] (Of course, this would also be a terrible diet because it lacks fruits and vegetables.) Most six- to nine-month-old infants consume approximately 1 quart of formula-based milk (with 400 IU of vitamin D) or infant formulas with even more vitamin D, as well as vitamin D-fortified cereals. They can easily receive more than the recommended 400 IU of vitamin D per day. In addition, it is not uncommon for pediatricians to prescribe an extra 400 IU of vitamin D per day.[276]

The requirement for vitamin D to ensure strong bones has led many individuals in our present health-conscious society to consume large supplements of vitamin D. Ironically, however, too much vitamin D can have the opposite effect because of the signals it sends to the body on how it uses calcium. The number one use for calcium in the body is for functioning of the blood. The second use for calcium is to build bones. Too much vitamin D sends the signal to the blood that it needs more calcium. The body takes this calcium from the bones or it takes it from the food we've eaten. Bones essentially are a reservoir for calcium to be used as needed. When there's not enough calcium in our food, the result is a bone reabsorption process. Bones become weaker as they provide the calcium to the blood, which is the top priority of the body in regards to calcium use. However, it is best to have enough calcium through food so that both the blood and the bones get the calcium they need. Excessive vitamin D stimulates bone reabsorption unless there is enough calcium in the diet.[270] This means drinking the equivalent of at least three glasses of milk a day.

When the extra calcium is in the blood because vitamin D has sent that signal to abandon the bone, that calcium has to go somewhere. It works its way into the artery cells. Too much calcium in the cell kills the cell. Those dead cells accumulate and calcify the arteries. Eventually this leads to the arteries being blocked and may cause a heart attack. Another possible outcome is that this calcification can lead to kidney failure.[277]

In addition to keeping track of our own vitamin D intake through either tablets or food additives, we can also be aware of the added amount of vitamin D originally added to meat products. Vitamin D added to the feed that animals eat carries over into the meat that we consume. Exactly how much vitamin D you take in depends on what cut of meat you're eating. For example, one FDA study[279] looked at chickens that ate commercial rations containing 4800 IU of vitamin D per day. This study found 4,086 IU in the skin, 363 IU in the breast muscle and 1725 IU in their liver. This same study found lean beef had 90 IU, liver sausage had 545 IU, and rockfish 2,700 per pound. Adults should have 400 IU of vitamin D per day, but the maximum depends on other factors such as how much calcium they have daily. Many people can get too much vitamin D.[276]

One study showed the amount of vitamin D in human blood was equivalent to the amount of vitamin D in the blood of pigs that had been fed a commercial ration high in vitamin D.[270] And if those people had also taken vitamin D supplements, the amounts in their blood would be even higher. Table 16 lists some selected sources of vitamin D and their percentages of the daily value (DV) or requirement.

Table 16: Selected food sources containing vitamin D[279]

Food	IU* per serving	Percent DV
Cod liver oil, 1 Tablespoon	1,360	340
Salmon, cooked, 3 ounces	360	90
Mackerel, cooked, 3 ounces	345	90
Tuna fish, canned in oil, 3 ounces	200	50
Sardines, canned in oil, drained, 1 ounce	250	70
Milk, nonfat, reduced fat, and whole, fortified, 1 cup	98	25
Margarine, fortified, 1 Tablespoon	60	15
Pudding, prepared from mix and made with vitamin D fortified milk, 1 serving	50	10
Ready-to-eat cereals fortified with 10% of the DV for vitamin D, to 1 cup servings (servings vary according to the brand)	40	10
Egg, 1 whole (vitamin D is found in egg yolk)	20	6
Liver, beef, cooked, 3 ounces	15	4
Cheese, Swiss, 1 ounce	12	4

*IU is international unit or one milligram. DV is daily value.

Antioxidants

The role of antioxidants in the body is:

• To prevent the improper metabolism of unsaturated fatty acids.

148

- To prevent eyesight problems such as macular degeneration.
- And who knows what else?

Exactly what the antioxidants contribute to health is still unknown. However, since they are often in health news, we are including them here. Antioxidants play a role in metabolism, the burning of certain calories. As you may recall from Chapter 2, unsaturated fatty acids are present both in vegetable oils and animal fats. If they are not metabolized properly, they are oxidized and that likely contributes to heart disease. These fats need to remain stable and in their original form. Antioxidants are believed to prevent that undesired oxidation so that fats stay in their original form. There are several types of antioxidants—one from vitamins and the other from flavonoids, the colored skin of fruit and vegetables, and the third from carotenoids. See Table 17 for a sample of flavonoid-containing foods.

Table 17: Antioxidants and their Sources in the Diet[280]

Type of Antioxidant	Typical Sources
Vitamins	C—Citrus fruits, like oranges and grapefruit; kiwi E—Soybean, wheat germ and corn oil B_6—Meat, eggs
Flavonoids	Fruits—blueberries, strawberries, blackberries, peaches, grapes, especially darker ones Vegetables—carrots, tomatoes, corn Herbs—rosemary, sage, thyme, oregano, and cloves Misc.—green tea, chocolate
Carotenoids	Yellow vegetables—carrots, squash Eggs

Some vitamins are considered antioxidants. Vitamins E and C worked as antioxidants in animals, but when tested in clinical studies of humans, were shown to be ineffective in preventing heart disease, and may even have the opposite effect of accelerating the oxidation leading to the development of atherosclerosis.[281] Vitamin B_6 has been shown recently to be an antioxidant in animals[282] but whether that will stand up in humans has yet to be shown.

Flavonoids are chemical components that color fruits, like blueberries, strawberries, and grapes, and vegetables like carrots, corn, and tomatoes. Often the darker the color, the more flavonoids present. For example, purple grapes have more than white grapes, and black raspberries have more than red raspberries. Red wine made from purple grapes is believed to be an antioxidant. Flavonoids are also present in green tea, chocolate, and herbs such as rosemary, sage, thyme, oregano, and cloves. They are believed to act as antioxidants in people, but this has not been definitely proven.[283] Some studies suggest that flavonoids may be helpful in alleviating symptoms of macular degeneration of the eye. Adult macular degeneration is the number one cause of blindness in individuals over 65 years old.

A synthetic antioxidant named BHT or butylated hydroxy toluene is used to prevent rancidity in food in the United States. BHT has been shown to be toxic and is not used in Europe but it is still used in the U.S., unfortunately. Something better than BHT is still unknown.

Carotenoids are also antioxidants, but specific names that may appear on food labels are lutein and zeaxanthin.[284] Yellow vegetables and egg yolks contain high amounts of these. Carotenoids protect the eyes from damage originating from ultraviolet rays of the sun. Studies have shown that a higher dietary intake of these two carotenoids lowers the risk for cataracts by up to 20% and age-related macular degeneration of the eye by up to 40%.[285] Carotenoids may also play a role in the prevention of some forms of cancer.[286]

While we do not know all the specific roles that antioxidants may play in our health, they nonetheless appear in foods that are good for us, such as fruits and vegetables. Therefore eating these is recommended.

CHAPTER 6 : Key Points

- Vitamins and minerals help carry out the processes required for you to live, such as stimulating your heart beat, keeping your blood flowing and providing structure to your bones.

- Remember, if you eat a balanced diet, you will have the vitamins and minerals that you need.

- You need not take supplements if you have a good diet. You may end up with too high a dose of a vitamin or a mineral if you do, and that may be harmful.

- If you have a poor diet with too much fat and sugar and not enough protein, fruits and vegetables, you may need supplements.
- It's better to get your vitamins and minerals naturally since the body absorbs them more easily

CHAPTER 7: Following the Government's "ChooseMyPlate" Will Not Guarantee A Healthy Diet: The Search for a Well-Balanced Diet

You need a balance of energy and nutrients in a your diet. The first step to eating right is to recognize the importance of all the components of a healthy diet. The second step is to eat those components in the right amounts. Did you know that the elements listed in Table 18 are all that is needed for a healthy diet?

Table 18: Components of a Healthy Diet

Components	Food Sources
Protein	Meat, eggs, dairy products such as milk, grains, beans, legumes, nuts, and seeds
Energy Sources	Carbohydrates including grains & starches; sugar including honey
Fat	Animal fat like butter and lard; vegetable fats like olive oil
Fiber	Grains, beans, fruits, and vegetables
Minerals	Calcium, magnesium, and trace minerals from grains, milk, meats, eggs, fruits, and vegetables
Vitamins and Antioxidants	A, D, E, K, C, and Bs from mostly fruits and vegetables, cereals, milk, meats, and eggs
Liquids	Water, milk, fruit juices

The food components listed in Table 18 also have specific functions in determining how cholesterol and fat are used in the body. Here's a quick review:

• Protein is needed to "carry" cholesterol and fat in the blood.

• Carbohydrates and fat are needed to provide the fuel that drives the muscle cells in the heart and the rest of the body. If not used for fuel, they are made into fat by the liver.

• Fibers are needed to help prevent the absorption of dietary sources of cholesterol from the digestive tract (the intestines). They move cholesterol through the intestinal tract faster so that less is absorbed.

- Minerals are needed to build bones. Traces of minerals along with proteins and vitamins are needed to build the thousands of enzymes that make cholesterol in the liver and bring the inert chemicals like sugar and fat in foods to "life."

- Liquids are needed because the majority of body mass is water: in men, it's about 72% and in women, it's 68%, due to a higher proportion of body fat. Liquids are needed to keep the blood fluid and flowing and as a component of all our body tissues. The "best" liquids contain nutrients as well; for example, milk contains calcium and protein, water contains some minerals, and fruit juices contain some minerals, fiber, and vitamins.

In the United States, the Department of Agriculture (USDA) takes the lead on setting standards for both what we should eat and the amount we should eat. It is the United States Food and Drug Administration (FDA) that oversees the safety of food items and drugs. To complete the picture, the Federal Trade Commission (FTC) oversees the claims made about the health benefits of various food products. It can be a confusing array of agencies involved in American diets. Another group, The National Academy of Sciences, Institute of Medicine acts as an advisory group to physicians and health professionals.

Let's begin with the USDA's recommendations about diets. They are illustrated in a schematic called "Choose my Plate".[287] You can look up your own diet recommendations, based on your age, gender, and activity level at www.choosemyplate.gov. This food guide is theoretically a good one to follow. It encourages eating grains and cereals as well as vegetables and fruits and dairy products. Protein sources such as meats and beans in moderate amounts are encouraged. Unfortunately, there are several major problems and myths with the recommendations:

- The recommendation on grains does not account for the nature of the grains currently available. It can be difficult to find whole grain foods that have not been over-processed thus removing the nutritional "value."

- The recommendations on protein treat all proteins as equal, when they are not. For example, beans and lean meats are presented as equal sources of protein, which they are not. Meat provides all the essential amino acids while beans do not.

- It gives preference to the linoleic acid in vegetable fats over linoleic acid in animal fats.

- It recommends skim milk over whole milk. Especially for children, whole milk contains "fats" that are needed to grow healthy bodies and brains. Drinking only skim milk does not provide these.

- It recommends calcium-fortified soy products as an alternative to dairy foods. However, soy products do not contain all of what dairy foods provide. Dairy products are complete proteins and soy products are not.

- It recommends cutting back on "hard" fats but does not differentiate between animal fats (which are good for you in moderation) and partially hydrogenated fats such as in margarine and shortenings, which are not good for you ever.

- It does not advise eliminating all partially hydrogenated trans fat from your diet, and it should! As manufacturers remove trans fats from their products, this point becomes moot.

- It doesn't recognize the actual nature of the American diet with so many non-nutritious (sugar and fat) energy sources of food leading to a need for more protein to carry the fat and cholesterol in the blood. Furthermore the extra calories we eat cause us to make more fat than is healthy for us.

Nature of Grains

As previously explained, the first problem concerns what grains and cereals are really like. Generally, whole cereals and whole grains are a good source of nutrients, including protein, minerals, and vitamins.[288-290] They are the basic food item between grower and consumer. However, cereals and grains in the U.S. are processed by milling (removing) the "natural" fat (wheat germ oil). This technology of grain milling was developed to produce white flour free of fat and parts of the wheat kernel, which would have given that white flour a gray appearance. After the B complex vitamins (vitamin B_1 thiamin, and vitamin B_2 riboflavin) became available they were added to white flour, along with iron. After 1938, niacin, and recently folic acid, were also added to white flour. The grains were then packaged for use at a later date. This manufacturing and packaging processing gets rid of important nutrients, resulting in an inferior product compared to the original "ingredients." Usually, the overall effect of food processing is to lessen the product's nutritional value rather than to increase it. The processing does, however, help to keep the product "stable" and thus "fresh" for the consumer.

It is a myth that "whole grain" bread is really whole grain, as it contains less protein than the "original" whole grain. Simply eating more of these "whole grains" will not provide the nutrition needed for a healthy diet. If you read cereal labels, you will see an attempt to return additional vitamins and minerals to the product. However, this may be done in a haphazard fashion with the result that it is possible to get too much of a vitamin, which can also be detrimental. As we explained earlier, vitamin D, which prevents rickets (bone deformations), in too great a quantity leads to atherosclerosis (hardening) of the arteries and heart disease.[266] An example of a positive vitamin additive is vitamin B_1 (thiamin), which prevents beriberi, another disease leading to death. When vitamin B_1 was added to rice, it cured the disease.[291] Polishing rice had removed the vitamin to the detriment of those consuming it. Overall, don't expect the grains we currently have available to provide you with enough of what is required for a healthy diet. You'll need to eat other foods since grains cannot provide enough nutrients including protein, vitamins and minerals.

Protein Sources

The second myth in the recommendations involves the sources of protein recommended by the USDA—lean meat, poultry, fish, beans, peas, nuts, and seeds. As noted earlier, one excellent source of inexpensive protein is seldom mentioned—eggs. Not all of these protein sources are equal in nutritional value. It is a myth to believe that one can simply substitute one protein source for another; for example, beans do not provide the same nutritional value to the body as a serving of meat or eggs and cannot be simply substituted for them in the diet. "Complete" proteins like meat and eggs contain eight essential amino acids, which are building blocks for proteins. The body makes 12 of those on its own, the other eight (nine for children) must be eaten from outside sources, i.e., the food you consume; you can't make those inside your body. All 20 are needed to build cells. Furthermore, you can't just eat any protein source and get those eight (nine for children) in the right amounts.[188] The food sources that do have all the essential ones are animal and fish food products. Those who eat vegetable

157

protein sources must have a mixture of various beans, peas, wheat, rice, etc., to gain all nine. Few people take the time or have the knowledge needed to do this.

A popular food for many people is pizza, which is made from wheat flour and a cheese source. The wheat flour is an incomplete protein even if it is a whole grain crust. The cheese source, if made from milk, is a complete protein. However, many of the cheeses are made from soy protein, which is also an incomplete protein. Pizza is also high in fat. Pizza is not a good source of protein and would lead to diet deficiencies.

Essential Nature of Both Animal and Vegetable Fats

It is a myth that vegetable fats are better than animal fats. As explained earlier, our bodies need both kinds of fats. Both are sources of essential fatty acids. Animal fat, i.e., saturated fat helps keep our organs fixed in place in our bodies. They also provide the saturated fat that combines with protein to carry to every cell in our bodies to provide energy for our daily tasks. Vegetable fats are largely composed of unsaturated fatty acids meaning that they are liquid at room temperature. We also need these fats for energy and to help keep our blood fluid. Thus both animal and vegetable fats are essential to a healthy diet.

Skim Versus Whole Milk

With diet conscious America, skim milk is being touted as the superior milk to drink. However, skim milk not only has fewer calories, but it has fewer nutrients. Adding Vitamin D and E to milk does not assure that it will be absorbed by the body. Fat is required to absorb those vitamins in the body. And that fat is easily provided in whole milk. This fat is especially important to children as it nourishes the formation of brain cells.

Dairy Milk Versus Soy Milk

It is not an equal exchange if you substitute one for the other and it should not be described as such. Dairy milk contains more fat than soy milk, but it also contains more healthy fats and it is a complete protein compared with the incomplete protein of soy products. Fortifying soy milk with calcium is a good step, but the calcium that naturally comes with milk is more nutritious and is more easily handled by the body.

Hydrogenated Fat

Here's the essence; as we have stated before, partially hydrogenated trans fats change the basic structure of cells and interfere with the process of keeping blood flowing smoothly. The FDA has banned trans fats although some are still in some food items on the shelf.

Trans fat can also accumulate with those small servings as well, and consumers may not even be aware they are eating it. Hydrogenated fat can be made trans free, but that will still not be nutritionally sound unless the essential fatty acids of omega-3 and omega-6 are added back into it. Trans fat from animal sources such as butter work differently in the body and do not create health risks; don't think twice about eating them (except if you eat too much of them!) Avoid eating anything with hydrogenated fat listed as one of the ingredients. The "plate" does recognize the need to keep trans fat consumption low and based on the new FDA ban, will undoubtedly include this.

Non-Nutritious Aspects of the American Diet

This one is not a myth—it is reality. The plate does not have any room for fats in our diets, suggesting we do not need much of these. Our current diet includes an over attachment to vegetable oils. These along with sugar make our food taste good, so to cut back on them is difficult. Sugar is only necessary as a supply of calories, or fuel, for our bodies. We should cut down on fats, oils and sugars to the recommended levels of no more than 35% of total calories. Oils and fats should not be cut out completely because they are necessary to provide both fluidity to our blood and structure to our bodies. Cutting down on calories will take some vigilance in part because many foods contain hidden sources of fats and sugars. Reading the labels is necessary.

We might do well to think of categorizing foods into those that add nutrients to our bodies (positive foods) and those that don't (negative foods). The negative foods are also considered empty calories; they bring only energy, but no necessary nutrients. Thus they bring our bodies more calories and often greater weight, but no real nutritional value. The foods on the "plate" for the most part emphasize the positive foods. But the reality of the American diet is that it contains many negative foods. These foods include candy, cakes, cookies, presweetened breakfast cereals, soft drinks, and processed foods of all kinds. The next chapter completes the picture of what you can do to eat a healthy diet.

Chapter 7. Key Points

• It is ironic that in the U.S. we have an abundance of food items at lower costs than most countries in the world. Yet, many of our food items have been stripped of some of their nutrients, or manufactured in a way to make them less nutritious, or even to contain "empty" calories.

• Unfortunately, more than half of our calories come from sugar, fats, and oils, when this should be about a third of our calories.

- The advice of the food plate is basically sound as far as it goes, but it does not go far enough.

CHAPTER 8: Preventing Heart Failure Through Better Nutrition: My Suggestions

There is no magic in a healthy diet, just a number of "ingredients": protein, carbohydrates, fat, fiber, vitamins, and minerals, and liquids eaten in the right amounts. Here is what I recommend that you eat.

Protein

• Eat a sufficient amount of protein! Protein is the building block of cells. The right amount depends on your weight, gender, activity level, and what else you're eating.

• Eat protein daily. You can't store it up to use a couple of days later.

• Eat protein sources with the right amounts of all the essential amino acids since your body must get those through food sources. If you eat eggs and animal products like meat, you don't need higher math to figure out the combinations since the essential ones are already there. If you eat vegetable proteins, check that you have the right combinations of amino acids. For example, beans and corn provide a good combination.

• Eat an egg a day in any form because it is a great source of protein and inexpensive. You'll find that it is quite filling and it has excellent nutritional properties. Don't worry about the cholesterol in eggs since so little of it is absorbed when eaten in a diet that contains grains, vegetables and fruit. Remember to eat both the white and the yellow part to get the maximum nutritional benefits.

• Eat other foods besides protein, in part so that protein is not used to provide the energy your body needs, but rather to provide the essential amino acids. Too much protein overtaxes your kidneys. You need nutrients from other sources like vegetable fat, animal fat, cereals, vegetables, fruits, minerals, and vitamins.

- If you eat food high in fat, like French fries, you need to eat food high in protein like chicken or hamburger to carry the fat in your system.

Fat

- Eat both animal and vegetable fat sources since they contain the needed essential fatty acids, omega-3 and omega-6. These must come from food sources since your body cannot make these essential fatty acids.

- Understand the ban on hydrogenated trans fats and do not eat them (unless trans free). Here's why:

  o They contribute excess calories to your diet and may make you heavier than you'd like.

  o They can change the basic fatty acid composition of your cells leading to atherosclerosis.

  o They inhibit the synthesis of prostacyclin that is needed to keep the blood flowing.

  o The amount can be cumulative.

  o You'll need to read the label to determine if a product has trans fat, since labeling mandates until now allowed the product to contain trans fat in a small amount and be labeled trans free if it was less than .5 grams per serving. Thus avoid any foods at present with hydrogenated or partially hydrogenated fat in the ingredient list since

164

they might contain trans fat. Hopefully in the near future manufacturers will sell trans free hydrogenated fat enriched with the essential fatty acids.

• Limit fat consumption to less than 30% of your caloric intake. If too much fat gets deposited in your body it can overwhelm various bodily systems. Remember that sugar and carbohydrates can turn into fat in the body if consumed in excess and not used for energy.

• Eat essential fatty acids that have more omega-6 than omega-3. They are present in nuts like walnuts, pecans, and almonds. They are also present in fish, seafoods, chicken and pork fat.

• Remember do not buy, let alone eat, anything with trans fat on the label until all foods are made trans free.

• Eat animal fats, including butter. They contain needed protein and essential fatty acids. Their trans fats work in positive ways in the body. Remember there are two sources of trans fats—those from hydrogenated vegetable oils, which are bad to eat, and those from natural animal fats like butter, which are good to eat in moderation.

• Avoid eating any commercially prepared food fried in fat because in the frying process the fat changes in composition to free radicals and 139 other unhealthy fats. If you do eat any of these fried foods, such as potato chips, French fries, etc., be sure you eat protein such as a hamburger, chicken, or seafood products along with it, to better carry the fat within your blood.

• If you fry your own foods, use the oil only once or twice, refrigerate it between uses, and then discard it. This is to avoid the oil becoming unhealthy. Again, make sure you eat protein with the fried food.

Carbohydrates

- Eat just enough carbohydrates to provide energy so that your body does not have to convert protein into energy and overtax your kidneys.
- It is better to eat complex carbohydrates (starches) than simple carbohydrates (sugar). An excess of sugar gets stored as fat. Starches take longer to break down in the body and are thus less likely to be stored as fat unless those starches are also eaten in surplus.
- Drink more water and fruit juices instead of soft drinks since fruit juices have some nutritional value.

Fibers

- Eat a variety of grains, fruits, and vegetables daily to provide both the soluble and insoluble fibers the body needs.
- Don't eat any one type of vegetable, fruit, or grain exclusively since no one category provides all the types of fibers your body needs.
- Don't overdo fibers because they may "wash" out necessary minerals.
- Make sure you eat other foods besides these since these are only part of a balanced diet.

Vitamins, Minerals, & Antioxidants

- If you eat a balanced diet, you will have the vitamins and minerals that you need, and it is not necessary to take vitamin and mineral supplements. It's better to get your vitamins and minerals naturally because the body absorbs them more easily.

- Include calcium-rich foods in your diet, such as milk, cheese, and leafy green vegetables. Calcium is important to build bones and also keep your heart pumping.

- Eat foods high in magnesium, such as natural whole grain cereals and vegetables and sea salt. Magnesium is needed to spark at least 100 processes in the body. Don't worry about overdoing the magnesium since it is water-soluble and the excess quickly passes out of our bodies in our urine.

- Make sure you have B vitamins—folic acid, vitamin B_6 and vitamin B_{12}—in your diet through natural sources such as meat products, milk products, and eggs. B vitamins are used to metabolize the proteins and fats properly.

- Try to limit the amount of vitamin D you ingest, by particularly avoiding food fortified with vitamin D and vitamin D supplements. Monitor how much vitamin D you eat by reading the labels of those products.

- Make sure you have enough calcium in your diet to counteract any "overdose" of vitamin D. Too much vitamin D increases the formation of atherosclerosis in the arteries, the leading cause of heart disease.

- Antioxidants are present naturally in our food such as fruits, fruit juices and vegetables, so please do not avoid them.

In general,

- Eat a balanced diet because it provides the ingredients your body needs to function.

- Cut back on calories from all sources including sugar (soft drinks), carbohydrates, and fats. Consuming too many calories is unhealthy and may lead to heart disease as well as other diseases due to obesity.
- Avoid eating between meals so that the body can use its fat in its fasting period.
- Retrain your eating habits to look for the positive foods and avoid the negative ones.

So What Could the Government Do? Recommendations

Try as you might to eat well, it could be advantageous to have the government make that process easier and thus ensure a healthy diet for everyone. People of all political persuasions can work together to lobby for better food-related regulations to benefit us all. After all, coming together over a meal is a universal activity.

Here are some things the government could do:

- Implement a number of FDA mandates to:
- Add magnesium to flour. This would help more people get the magnesium they need daily.
- Add vitamin B_6 and B_{12} to flour since many people, particularly teenagers, are not likely to get enough of it in their diets.
- Stop food producers from putting vitamin D into new food products. There is already too much vitamin D in the diet, and it is easy to get through sunlight and other fortified foods.
- Substantially reduce the amount of vitamin D being put into animal feeds and remove the vitamin D entirely from the feed several days before the animal goes to market. This would help reduce

the amount of vitamin D that is in animal food products.

- Restrict the over-the-counter sales of vitamin D as a nutritional supplement. Most people do not need additional vitamin D.

- Have the FDA provide money to analyze food for content of vitamin D; at present this is not done. This would allow people to figure out how much vitamin D they are consuming and to adjust their diets accordingly.

- Have the FDA mandate a label listing the amounts of each essential amino acid in a food item. This may help those who are vegetarian or vegan to have a more nutritious diet.

- Encourage the FDA to require restaurants to (a) set standards for freshness and (b) test frying fat frequently for its freshness. This would lead to healthier food for the consumer. Testing is mandated in Germany.

- Contact the FDA (www.fda.gov) with your concerns.

- Encourage all groups that give diet recommendations, such as the USDA, to change their recommendations to include eating one egg a day. This would be an inexpensive way of getting more essential amino acids into the diet.

- Pass legislation to keep farmland as farmland. Because we need both animal and vegetable sources of protein and fat, the government should not allow land that is currently cultivated for crops to go to other uses. Remember very little land is actually good for cultivating crops. There is a negative, long- range impact if farmland is lost to the development of urban areas.

- Increase funding for basic research. Expecting the pharmaceutical companies to fund basic research programs is counter-productive. Their mission is to make money for their shareholders by providing products that benefit their bottom line. Instead, laboratories supported by taxpayers should conduct basic research. For example in Germany, the government-funded Max Planck Institutes conduct such research.

Our food distribution system makes it possible for us to eat fruits, vegetables, dairy products, eggs, and meat at any time of the year. Now we have to get ourselves to eat them in the right amounts! Some people want the magic diet to maintain weight and avoid heart disease. It seems that some believe that managing cholesterol is the magic needed, but I hope I have convinced you that it is not. The magic is already operating: how the body takes ordinary food and converts it into fuel to make the body function.

Key Points: So What Do I Eat?

Here's my typical diet:

- For breakfast: An egg, cooked whole wheat grains and oatmeal served with several kinds of fruit, including a banana and those with a colored skin, and topped with milk, a few walnuts, pecans or almonds, and yogurt. Orange juice and milk.
- For lunch at home: Sometimes, vegetables or vegetable soup that uses up any vegetable leftovers. A piece of whole wheat bread with cheese. Fruit. Milk. During my days at the Burnside Research Lab I took a piece of whole wheat bread that my wife made, with cheese and an apple.

- For dinner: Meat or fish prepared under the broiler. Baked potato. Some fresh or frozen vegetables. Lettuce salad. Fruit. A cup of tea. I have a nutritious dinner using the broiler, microwave, and stove.

- I still exercise every day.

- I weigh myself weekly and if I am gaining weight, I eat less for the next 3-4 days. (That is the best way to lose weight; you'll be surprised to note that you have lost a pound!) If I am losing weight, I treat myself to a dessert of ice cream or cherry pie.

About the Authors
Fred Kummerow, Ph.D., with Jean Kummerow, Ph.D.

In writing this book, I've used my vantage point as a biochemist and food scientist who has worked in this field for over seven decades, beginning during the Great Depression in the late 1930s. My major focus has been research into heart disease and the impact of diet on that disease. When I began my work, there was little research in that field. Now just pick up a newspaper and you'll see a different story. I am currently 99 years old and still find basic research into what people eat and how that affects heart disease fascinating, and I plan to work in the field as long as I am funded.

I was born in Berlin, Germany in 1914. There was very little food available during my early years and my Mother used to put me and my brother to bed during the day and entertained us rather than let us run around burning calories we didn't have. We emigrated to the US in 1923. We also faced food shortages during the Depression but we got some government rations that helped us out. Perhaps this lack of food as a child steered me into food science as an adult!

I was given a chemistry set when I was 12 by a relative and was fascinated. I attended Milwaukee's Boys Technical School because they had a three-year chemistry course at the time. I enjoyed learning and have kept learning my entire life. I began college in Milwaukee in 1933 at the University of Wisconsin Extension Division night school, and attended for three years while working 48 hours a week at a wholesale drug company. In 1936, I transferred to the Department of Chemistry at the University of Wisconsin in Madison.

I participated in a National Youth Administration (NYA) program that enabled students like me with no personal or family resources to attend college. In 1939 I became a graduate student in the Department of Biochemistry at the University of Wisconsin in Madison. My Master's degree research[279] showed how important, even how essential, it is to consume vegetable oil to give birth to healthy children. This oil contains unsaturated fatty acids (and I hope by now you know what those are!). Over 40 years later, this study was listed as a classic in nutrition.[280]

My Ph.D. research[281] involved identifying the chemistry of a factor in the blood (linoleic acid) that keeps the blood from clotting in the arteries and veins. This is a particularly important factor in today's heart disease research since that clotting affects the blood flow from the heart.

In 1943, I left for a position at Clemson University in Clemson, South Carolina, for a National Research Council-sponsored study on the disease pellagra. Research at the University of Wisconsin in 1938 had already discovered that a deficiency of a vitamin called niacin was responsible for the development of that disease. In the southeastern part of the U.S. at that time, a typical diet for some people consisted of corn, often in the form of grits (ground corn), and pork fat. They did not eat red meat, eggs, or dairy products, all of which in the diet would have prevented pellagra. Even in 1942, some 2,000 people died annually of that disease in the U.S. Public and private groups came together to fund a project to see what could be done to prevent pellagra. Since corn was a major component of the diet there, my first job was to find how corn could be fortified by niacin in order to prevent this disease.

At that time, many people grew their own corn and took it to a mill to be ground into grits. The trick was to get the niacin and other nutrients including iron and vitamins into the corn in a way that the consumer would accept; in its pure form, the niacin made the grits look "dirty." We had a macaroni manufacturer make a mixture with the necessary iron and vitamins baked into it. The macaroni was broken up to look like corn, taken to the mills in the area, and added to

174

the corn. Since it then looked like corn and didn't wash out, the consumers left it in their grits. The procedure worked well.

The next step then was to show manufacturers that the grits were actually fortified and that they could do this themselves in a simple way with fortified macaroni. I stained the iron in the formula with a chemical that made it blue and then baked it into the macaroni. The blue-colored macaroni proved that the niacin was still there. Thus we could show large manufacturers of corn grits that the fortification process worked.

The corn grit millers were invited to a meeting in Chicago hosted by the National Research Council, a government agency. After considerable discussion, they agreed to add niacin to the corn grits they marketed in the southern U.S. In just three years, there were only 12 deaths from pellagra in the U.S. Thus, I know firsthand the impact of adding necessary ingredients to food and the difference that makes in people's lives. I know that a vitamin lacking in the diet can kill someone, and I know this can be changed.

I left Clemson in 1945 for a position in the chemistry department at Kansas State University in Manhattan, Kansas, where I established a basic research program in lipid chemistry. Lipid chemistry is simply the chemistry of fats (e.g., butter, margarine, lard, vegetable oils, trans fats, etc.). Some of my work at Kansas State involved the technology of storing foods, especially those containing fat.

Food with certain fats goes "bad" or rancid quickly. This issue was particularly important during World War II and its aftermath when the American Armed Forces were scattered worldwide. The food provided to them was sometimes exposed to extreme heat or intense cold, so it had to be processed in a way to keep it fresh.

The Army Quartermaster Corp granted contracts to various universities to develop methods to keep food items edible during extreme conditions. I had such a contract. The

Army Quartermaster Corp required reports, which were marked restricted. The reports were circulated to all the contract sites and also to food manufacturing companies who then used the information to furnish edible and tasty food products to the Armed Forces.

I was part of a project to improve the quality of frozen turkeys and chickens. Essentially our solution was to change the standard poultry diet to one that prevented the fat in the meat from turning rancid, leaving an acceptable taste[282] when it was consumed. I received a citation for this work from the Army Quartermaster Corp in January 1948. Ultimately this research made the sale of frozen chickens and turkeys possible in grocery stores today.

I was invited to move my lipid research program to the University of Illinois in Urbana, Illinois, in 1950, where I have been ever since. Several events shaped my career there. As research was important to the military during World War II, it made sense after the war to continue funding research projects to help the civilian population as well. In 1948 the U.S. Congress created the National Institutes of Health (NIH) and made research funds available on a variety of topics, including diet and health.

The NIH was mandated to fund research on cancer and other diseases, but only a few million dollars per year were allocated for heart research until after President Eisenhower's heart attack in 1955. Since then billions of dollars have gone into heart research. However, people are still developing heart disease and it is the leading cause of death in the U.S. and in every developed country of the world.

With money available from NIH grants to study heart disease, I began to work in that field. The effect of cholesterol on heart disease was one avenue of study and was the one I followed. Almost everyone now has heard of cholesterol and its possible link to heart disease, with recommendations (I disagree with) to cut back on eating

176

cholesterol-containing foods such as eggs and meat, and saturated fats in foods like butter.

For 50 years, cholesterol has been considered the number one factor in heart disease in spite of the 50 years of research that has not shown this conclusively. My research even suggests that this focus on lowering cholesterol has led to a wrong course of action. Cholesterol that has not been used properly by the body is the problem rather than cholesterol in the food itself or even the cholesterol in one's blood.

My recommendations on what to eat are designed to minimize the impact of cholesterol not used appropriately by the body. These suggestions are for readily available foods to eat in the right combination to lower naturally the body's inappropriate use of cholesterol.

A second factor during my career at the University of Illinois was to study the biochemistry of trans fats in foods. Trans fats are now in the news as a health concern. I began documenting my concerns about the negative effects of trans fats in 1957.[21] I hope this book has convinced you that these are unhealthy. I am gratified that the FDA has proposed measures to ban all manufactured trans fats from our food.

I want to share my 75+ years of laboratory research with you. Looking back, I have been directly involved in food-related research since 1936. I have been an expert witness on cholesterol for several hearings before the Federal Trade Commission,[202,203] and have provided a report to a U.S. Senate hearing on nutrition and the biochemistry of cholesterol.

I have authored or coauthored close to 500 peer-reviewed scientific papers, edited two books, and contributed chapters to six books on the role of trans fat and cholesterol in heart disease. I have documented the dangers of trans fats since the late 1950s.

I have been in two television documentaries on trans fats, which have been aired in Canada and Great Britain, but not in the United States. A crew of five members from Canada spent a week in Urbana in 1979, and I recently received an e-mail from one of them, Robert Fripp, commenting on how ahead of the issue we were.

Both documentaries would have alerted Americans to the undesirable presence of trans fats 20 years before the FDA expressed interest in trans fats. Publications since 1957 in peer-reviewed international and American scientific journals co-authored with physicians at a local hospital have documented my concerns about the effects of trans fat. These studies have shown that arteries change in composition (leading to blockages) in patients with heart disease and that these changes were not related to dietary cholesterol or the concentration of cholesterol in the blood.

Since the late 1970s, I have called attention to the imbalance of nutrients in the American diet that has led to obesity. It is hard for people to avoid hidden fats and calories in the American diet.

The editor of a journal named Magnesium Research stated that approximately 60-70% of papers presented in international magnesium symposiums were related to clinical medicine and about 30% to clinical nutrition. In a 1995 issue, it stated, "We are introducing Professor Kummerow who is one of the very few researchers in basic medical sciences. Dr. Kummerow has published more than 300 papers during his long lasting research career. Although it is unable to know all these papers, recent publications show that his research has been focused mainly toward the study of relationship between lipid metabolism and atherosclerosis. Since 1989, Dr. Kummerow's group has reported many outstanding research achievements by using advanced biochemical methods. These accomplishments are worthy of attention in a sense that they provided biochemical proof needed for the clinical observations and speculations made by many Magnesium researchers."[16]

Funding for research is always a challenge for scientists. For example, in 1985, I submitted a program project grant proposal on the causes of heart disease to the NIH, which involved 15 professors in five different colleges at the University of Illinois. We had a team of 15 NIH site visitors spend a day with us listening to how we wanted to work together trying to solve what causes heart disease. When I called Dr. Louis Oulette, the NIH representative, to ask how we fared, he said, "You were ten years ahead of the site visit team. You can only be ahead two to three years to get funded".

Dr. Claude Lefant, director of the National Lung and Blood Institute, at the time, urged me to try again. The next time we were approved for funding, but the funds were no longer there. Throughout the years, my research has been funded first through government grants and then more and more through private sources, as government funds are becoming more difficult to obtain. I am presently trying again to put together a multi-disciplinary team funded through private sources to focus on the causes of heart disease. Heart disease is too large a problem for any one researcher to solve, yet every person who lives long enough has some degree of heart disease.

I am a member of a number of professional organizations and have been named a fellow (a recognition of competence) in the American Association for the Advancement of Science, the American College of Nutrition, the American Society of Nutritional Sciences, the International Society for Atherosclerosis, the American Heart Association Council on Arteriosclerosis, Thrombosis and Vascular Biology, and the Council on Clinical Cardiology. I have been president of the Illinois Heart Association, a member of the subcommittee on fats of the American Heart Association, and have visited medical and university research laboratories the world over. I am also a member of a yahoo-based group called The International

Network of Cholesterol Skeptics (THINCS). So much for my professional qualifications!

Personally, I knew enough to eat right and I exercised! I practiced what I preached. What could go wrong? When I was 89 years old, I told Dr. Scott Cook, the heart surgeon I had been collaborating with on research at Carle Hospital in Urbana, Illinois, that I sometimes felt a tightening around my collarbone after a hurried walk, but not during my daily quarter-mile swim. He suggested an echocardiogram, the results of which showed a lack of blood circulation in the upper left chamber of my heart. A cardiac catheterization indicated major blockage in the left coronary artery; old age had caught up with me.

Even though I never had a heart attack, Dr. Cook recommended coronary artery bypass grafting (CABG) surgery, which I had on March 23, 2004. Now I'm back exercising without that tightening feeling in my collarbone and back working at my research on diet and heart disease with even more interest.

Jean Kummerow is my daughter who has a Ph.D. in Counselling and Student Personnel Psychology from the University of Minnesota and her bachelor's from Grinnell College in Iowa. She is an applied psychologist who uses psychological principles primarily in organizational and community settings to help people identify work they find satisfying and to develop better working relationships through improved communication, decision-making and teamwork.

A particular specialty of hers is the Myers-Briggs Type Indicator® instrument, and she trains professionals internationally in its interpretation, writes application materials on how to use it, and applies it with individuals and groups. She is also on contract as a leadership coach and coordinator to the Blandin Foundation's Community Leadership Program, a program to strengthen Minnesota's small towns by teaching leadership skills. Her role in this book was to attempt to translate scientific principles into simple language, but she admits that she at times had to give up. We hope what we did together will be clear enough for you to understand the nutritional principles and begin to eat as well as your body deserves.

For more on the author, visit:
http://www.spacedoc.com/fred-kummerow-bio

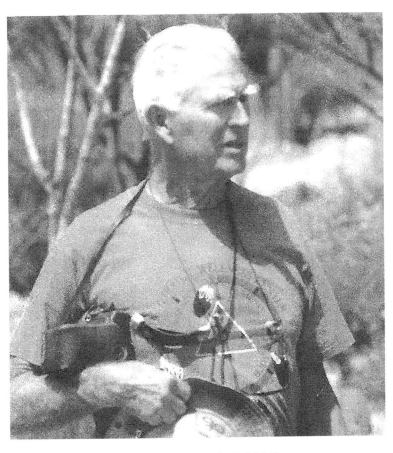

H.B. Wallace (1915-2005)
A longtime friend and supporter of my work.

Acknowledgements

I owe a debt of gratitude to the 57 graduate students, 32 post doctorates, and 17 visiting professors that I have been privileged to work with from 1945 to the present. I am grateful to my research colleagues, Dr. Qi Zhou and Dr. M. M. Mahfouz, who have worked with me for the last 25 years.

Through my 65 year research career, I have received funding from the Illinois Heart Association, the American Heart Association (AHA), the National Institutes of Health (NIH), the National Science Foundation (NSF), and the United States Department of Agriculture (USDA). Several companies and associations provided support early in my career and these include the Borden Company, Armour and Company, Swift, Archer Daniels Midland (ADM), Quaker Oats, The National Livestock and Meat Board, the National Dairy Council, and The Pure Milk Association. Several individuals and foundations have supported my work, and these include Ethel Burnsides, who provided funds for the construction of the Burnsides Research Laboratory and willed oil revenue money to the University of Illinois Foundation for my research; The Wallace Research Foundation; the John R. and Verna L. Hildebrand Foundation; and the Weston A. Price Foundation. And of course, I thank my cardiac surgeon, Dr. Scott Cook.

I've had numerous assistants and assistance with both editions including Yan Shen, Megan Leffelman, Katy Stewart, Arlene West, Leatrice Potter, Lou Ann Carper, Marisol Chirinos, Anita Gentille, and Chris Masterjohn.

Note: Permissions for the use of the figures and tables have been granted. Reference to the original published literature is indicated.

References

1. Lodish H. Molecular Cell Biology 5ed: W.H. Freeman and Co.; 2004.
2. Lehninger A. Biochemistry. New York, NY: Worth Publishers Inc.; 1970.
3. Kummerow FA. Metabolism of Lipids as Related to Atherosclerosis. Springfield, IL: Charles C. Thomas; 1965.
4. Kummerow FA. Hypothesis: possible role of magnesium and calcium in the development of structure and function of the plasma membrane in mammalian cells and in human diseases. J Am Coll Nutr. 1992;11:410-425.
5. Belkhadir Y, Chory J. Brassinosteroid signaling: a paradigm for steroid hormone signaling from the cell surface. Science. 2006;314:1410-1411.
6. Kritchevsky D. Cholesterol. New York: John Wiley & Sons, Inc.; 1958.
7. Krebs H. Biography: The Nobel Foundation; 2005.
8. Bloch K. The Biological Synthesis of Cholesterol. J Biol Chem. 1964;1:79-98.
9. Kokatnur M, Rand NT, Kummerow FA. Effect of the energy to protein ratio on serum and carcass cholesterol levels in chicks. Circ Res. 1958;6:424-431.
10. Geer JC, McGill Jr. HC, Strong JP. The fine structure of human atherosclerotic lesions. Am J Pathol. 1961;38:263-287.
11. Dietschy JM. Regulation of Cholesterol Metabolism in Man and in Other
Species. Klin Wochenschr. 1984;62:338-345.
12. Grundy SM, Ahrens EH. Measurements of cholesterol turnover, synthesis and absorption in man, carried out by isotope kinetic and sterol balance methods. J Lipid Res. 1969;10:91-107.
13. Kandutsch AA, Chen HW. Inhibition of sterol synthesis in cultured mouse cells by 7alpha-hydroxycholesterol, 7beta-hydroxycholesterol, and 7-ketocholesterol. J Biol Chem. 1973;248:8408-8417.
14. Kandutsch AA, Chen HW. Regulation of sterol synthesis in cultured cells by oxygenated derivatives of cholesterol. J Cell Physiol. 1975;85:415-424.
15. Fournier NC. Lipid Metabolism in the Normoxic and Ischaemic Heart. New York: Springer-Verlag; 1987.
16. Editor. The Magnesium Researchers: Fred A. Kummerow. Current Concepts in Magnesium Research. 1995;7:14-15.

17. Page I. The Chemistry of Lipids as Related to Atherosclerosis. Springfield, IL: AR Thomas; 1958.

18. DeBakey ME, Dietrich EB, Garrett HE, McCutchen JJ. Surgical Treatment of Cerebrovascular Disease. Postgrad Med J. 1967;42:218-226.

19. DeBakey ME, Crawford ES, Cooley DA, Morris GC, Jr. Surgical Considerations of Occlusive Disease of Innominate, Carotoid, Subclavian, and Cerebral Arteries. Ann Surg. 1959;149:690-710.

20. Kummerow FA, Przybylski R, Wasowicz E. Changes in arterial membrane lipid composition may precede growth factor influence in the pathogenesis of atherosclerosis. Artery. 1994;21:63-75.

21. Johnston PV, Johnson OC, Kummerow FA. Occurrence of trans fatty acids in human tissue. Science. 1957;126:698-699.

22. Kummerow FA, Mahfouz MM, Zhou Q, Cook LS. 27-Hydroxycholesterol causes remodeling in endothelial cell membrane lipid composition comparable to remodeling in the failed vein grafts of CABG patients. Life Sci. 2006;78:958-963.

23. Kummerow FA. Nutrition imbalance and angiotoxins as dietary risk factors in coronary heart disease. Am J Clin Nutr. 1979;32:58-83.

24. Anitschkow NN. A History of Experimentation on Arterial Atherosclerosis in Animals. In: Blumenthal HT, ed. Cowdry's Arteriosclerosis: A Survey of the Problem. 2 ed. Springfield, IL: Charles C. Thomas; 1967:21-44.

25. Mahfouz MM, Kummerow FA. Cholesterol-rich diets have different effects on lipid peroxidation, cholesterol oxides, and antioxidant enzymes in rats and rabbits. J Nutr Biochem. 2000;11:293-302.

26. Grundy SM, Havel R, Howard E. The evolution of lipoprotein analysis. J Clin Invest. 2004;114:1034-1037.

27. Lindgren FT, Nichols AV. In Plasma Proteins. Vol 2. New York: Academic Press Inc.; 1960.

28. Morrisett JD, Gotto AM. Lipoprotein Structure and Metabolism. Physiol Rev. 1976;56:256-259.

29. Fredrickson DS. The Inheritance of High Density Lipoprotein Deficiency (Tangier Disease). J Clin Invest. 1964;43:228-236.

30. Grundy SM, al. e. National Cholesterol Education Program Expert Panel on Detection, Evaluation, and Treatment of High Blood Cholesterol in Adults. Circulation. 2002;106:3145-3421.

31. Association AH. American Heart Association, What Your Numbers Mean; 2006.
32. Grundy SM. Cholesterol metabolism in man. West J Med. 1978;128:13-25.
33. Lupton JR. Dietary Reference Intakes: Energy, Carbohydrate, Fiber, Fatty Acids, Cholesterol, Protein, and Amino Acids - Part 1. Vol 25. Washington D.C.: Institute of Medicine of the National Academies; 2002.
34. Flynn MA, Nolph GB, Osio Y, et al. Serum lipids and eggs. J Am Diet Assoc. 1986;86:1541-1548.
35. Pownall HJ, Jackson RL, Roth RI, Gotto AM, Patsch JR, Kummerow FA. Influence of an atherogenic diet on the structure of swine low density lipoproteins. J Lipid Res. 1980;21:1108-1115.
36. Mahley RW, Weisgraber KH, Innerarity T, Brewer HB, Jr., Assmann G. Swine lipoproteins and atherosclerosis. Changes in the plasma lipoproteins and apoproteins induced by cholesterol feeding. Biochemistry. 1975;14:2817-2823.
37. Jackson RL, Morrisett JD, Pownall HJ, et al. Influence of dietary trans-fatty acids on swine lipoprotein composition and structure. J Lipid Res. 1977;18:182- 190.
38. McGill HC, Jr. The relationship of dietary cholesterol to serum cholesterol concentration and to atherosclerosis in man. Am J Clin Nutr. 1979;32:2664
39. Truswell AS. Diet in the pathogenesis of ischaemic heart disease. Postgrad Med J. 1976;52:424-432.
40. Groves B. Statins: Saviours of Mankind, or Expensive Scam? Second Opinions; 2004.
41. Brensike JF, Levy RI, Kelsey SF, et al. Effects of therapy with cholestyramine on progression of coronary arteriosclerosis: results of the NHLBI Type II Coronary Intervention Study. Circulation. 1984;69:313-324.
42. Folkers K, Langsjoen P, Willis R, et al. Lovastatin decreases coenzyme Q levels in humans. Proc Natl Acad Sci U S A. 1990;87:8931-8934.
43. Mohr D, Bowry VW, Stocker R. Dietary supplementation with coenzyme Q10 results in increased levels of ubiquinol-10 within circulating lipoproteins and increased resistance of human low-density lipoprotein to the initiation of lipid peroxidation. Biochim Biophys Acta. 1992;1126:247-254.
44. Crofts AR. The cytochrome bc1 complex: function in the context of structure. Annu Rev Physiol. 2004;66:689-73.

45. Zhou Q, Zhou Y, Kummerow FA. High-dose lovaststin decreased basal prostacyclin production in cultured endothelial cells. Prostaglandins &. Other Lipid Mediators. 89(2009)1-7.

46. Lambert V. The Worrying 32 Billion Dollar Wonder Drug: World Institute of Natural Health Sciences; 2007.

47. Lipitor: atorvastatin calcium tablets *Circulation*; 2006.

48. Tawakol A, et al. Intensification of Statin Therapy Results in a Rapid Reduction in Atherosclerotic Inflammation.Results of a Multi-Center FDG-PET/CT Feasibility study. JAM Coll Cardiol, 2013 May 30. pii:so735-1097(13)02082-2. doi:10.1016/j. JACC.2013.04.066

49. Pedersen TR, Kjekshus J, Berg K, et al. Randomised trial of cholesterol lowering in 4444 patients with coronary heart disease: the Scandinavian Simvastatin Survival Study (4S). 1994. Atheroscler Suppl. 2004;5:81-87.

50. Hobbs FD. Type-2 diabetes mellitus related cardiovascular risk: new options for interventions to reduce risk and treatment goals. Atheroscler Suppl. 2006;7:29- 32.

51. Mahfouz M, Zhou Q, Kummerow FA. Inhibition of prostacyclin release by cigarette smoke extract in endothelial cells is not related to enhanced superoxide generation and NADPH-oxidase activation. J Environ Pathol Toxicol Oncol. 2006;25:585-595.

52. Nilsson et al.No connection between the level of expsition to statins in the population and the incidence/mortality of acute myocardial infarction: An ecological study on Sweden's municipalities. Journal of Negative Results in BioMedicine 2011, 10:6. http://www.jnrbm.com/content/10/1/6.

53. Endo A. The discovery and development of HMG-CoA reductuase iinhibitors. J Lipid Res 1992;33:1569-82

54. Havel RJ, Rapaport E. Management of primary hyperlipidemia. N Engl J Med 1995;332:1491-8

55. MAAS Investigators. Effects of simvastatin on coronary atheroma: the multicenter anti-atheroma study (MAAS). Lancet 1994;344:633-8

56. NCEP Expert Panel on Detection, Evaluation, and Treatment of HighBlood Cholesterol in Adults. Summary of the second report of the national cholesterol education program (NCEP) expert panel on detection, evaluation, and treatment of high blood cholesterol in adults (Adult treatment panel II). JAMA 1993;269:3015-23

57. Levine L. Statins stimulated arachidonic acid release and prostaglandin I2 production in rat liver cells. Lipids Health Dis 2003:2.

58. Hrboticky N, Tang I, Zimmer B, Lux I, Weber PC. Lovastatin increases arachidonic acid levels and stimulates thromboxane synthesis in human liver and monocytic cell lines. J Clin Invest 1994;93:195-203.

59. Duffy D, Rader DJ. Emerging therapies targeting high-density lipoprotein metabolism and reverse cholesterol transport. Circulation. 2006;113:1140-1150.

60. Libby P. The forgotten majority: unfinished business in cardiovascular risk reduction. J Am Coll Cardiol. 2005;46:1225-1228.

61. Pilgeram L. Atherogenesis: Historical perspective biochemical mechanism current statue. Presentation lecture series sponsored by the Phillips Medication Education Fund; 2000.

62. Kummerow FA. Nutritional Imbalance and Angiotoxins as Dietary Risk Factors in Coronary Heart Disease. Am. J. Clin. Nutr. 1979; 32:58-83.

63. Kamio A, Kummerow FA, Taura S, Tokuyasu K, Cleveland JC. Ultrastructure of Human Aorta: Cellular Composition of Diffuse Intimal Thickening. Med. Bull. Fukuoka Univ. 1976;4:15-28.

64. Kamio A, Taguchi T, Shiraishi M, et al. Mast cells in human aorta. Paroi Arterielle. 1979;5:125-136.

65. Takagi T, Leszczynski D, Toda T, Kummerow F, Nishimori I. Ultrastructure of human umbilical artery and vein. Characterization and quantification of lipid laden cells. Acta Pathol Jpn. 1985;35:1047-1055.

66. Takagi T, Toda T, Leszczynski D, Kummerow F. Ultrastructure of aging human umbilical artery and vein. Acta Anat (Basel). 1984;119:73-79.

67. Taura S, Taura M, Tokuyasu K, Kamio A, Kummerow FA. Ultrastructure of Human Thoracic Aorta Obtained at Elective Coronary Bypass Surgery. Artery. 1977;6:529-541.

68. Huang WY, Kummerow FA. Esterification of palmitic acid in swine aortic microsomes. Biochem Med. 1978;20:371-377.

69. Kamio A, Huang WY, Cho BH, Imai H, Kummerow FA. Aortic intimal changes in aging swine. Paroi Arterielle. 1977;4:27-43.

70. Kamio A, Huang WY, Imai H, Kummerow FA. Mitotic structures of aortic smooth muscle cells in swine and in culture: paired cisternae. J Electron Microsc (Tokyo). 1977;26:29-40.

71. Kummerow FA, Mizuguchi T, Arima T, Cho B, Hang W. The influence of three sources of dietary fats and cholesterol on lipid composition of swine serum lipids and aorta tissue. Artery. 1978;4:360-384.

72. Moriuchi A, Imai H, Kummerow FA. Ultrastructural studies of coronary arterial intima. I. Intimal cell nest and serofibrinous insudation in 6-month-old swine. Exp Mol Pathol. 1982;36:19-33.

73. Taura S, Taura M, Imai H, Kummerow F. Coronary Atherosclerosis in Normacholesterolemic Swine. . Artery. 1978;4:395-407.

74. Taura S, Taura M, Imai H, Kummerow FA. Morphological alteration of aortic wall and mitotic cells after complete endothelial loss induced by repeated balloon denudation of swine aorta. Tohoku J Exp Med. 1979;129:25-39.

75. Taura S, Taura M, Kummerow FA. Human Arterio- and Atherosclerosis: Identical to that in a 6 and 36 Month Old Swine Fed a Corn Diet Free of Cholesterol and Saturated Fat. Artery. 1978;4:100-106.

76. Taura S, Taura M, Kummerow FA, Kamio A, Takebayashi S. Mitotic structure of aortic intimal cells induced by mechanical injury in swine. Acta Pathol Jpn. 1978;28:555-564.

77. Toda T, Leszczynski DE, Kummerow FA. Degenerative changes in endothelial and smooth muscle cells from aging swine ductus arteriosus and venosus. Am J Anat. 1981;160:37-49.

78. Toda T, Mahfouz MM, Kummerow FA. Influence of dietary fats on ultrastructure and fatty acid composition of swine arterial tissue. Acta Pathol Jpn. 1984;34:935-945.

79. Huang WY, Kamio A, Yeh S-J, Kummerow F. The influence of vitamin D on plasma and tissue lipids and atherosclerosis in swine. Artery. 1977;3:439-455.

80. Taura S, Taura M, Imai H, Kummerow FA, Tokuyasu K, Cho SB. Ultrastructure of cardiovascular lesions induced by hypervitaminosis D and its withdrawal. Paroi Arterielle. 1978;4:245-259.

81. Taura S, Taura M, Kamio A, Kummerow FA. Vitamin D-induced coronary atherosclerosis in normolipemic swine: comparison with human disease. Tohoku J Exp Med. 1979;129:9-16.

82. Toda T, Leszczynski DE, Kummerow FA. The role of 25-hydroxy-vitamin D3 in the induction of atherosclerosis in swine and rabbit by hypervitaminosis D. Acta Pathol Jpn. 1983;33:37-44.

83. Toda T, Mizoe A, Ohishi K, Toda Y, Kummerow FA. Coronary Arerial Lesions in Swine Fed Supplemental Vitamin D with Skimmed Milk Powder. J Jpn Atheroscler Soc. 1986;13:1475-1480.

84. Toda T, Toda Y, Kummerow FA. Coronary arterial lesions in piglets from sows fed moderate excesses of vitamin D. Tohoku J Exp Med. 1985;145:303-310.

85. Stein EV, Glueck CJ, Morrison JA. Coronary risk factors in the young. Annu Rev Med. 1981;32:601-613.

86. Ito M, Cho BH, Kummerow FA. Effects of a dietary magnesium deficiency and excess vitamin D3 on swine coronary arteries. J Am Coll Nutr. 1990;9:155- 163.

87. Kawamura K, Kummerow FA. Effect of magnesium deficiency on 15-hydroxyeicosatetraenoic acid in cultured human umbilical arterial endothelial cells. Magnes Res. 1992;5:109-113.

88. Kawano H, Yokoyama S, Smith TL, Nishida HI, Taguchi T, Kummerow FA. Effect of magnesium on secretion of platelet-derived growth factor by cultured human umbilical arterial endothelial cells. Magnes Res. 1995;8:137-144.

89. Kummerow FA, Mahfouz M, Zhou Q. Cholesterol metabolism in human umbilical arterial endothelial cells cultured in low magnesium media. Magnes Res. 1997;10:355-360.

90. Kummerow FA. New Insights between Magnesium and lipid status. In: Palpern MJ, Durlach J, eds. Current Research in Magnesium. John Libbey and Co.; 1996:59-61.

91. Mahfouz MM, Kummerow FA. Effect of magnesium deficiency on delta 6 desaturase activity and fatty acid composition of rat liver microsomes. Lipids. 1989;24:727-732.

92. Mahfouz MM, Smith TL, Kummerow FA. Decreased uptake of low density lipoprotein by LLC-PK cells cultured at low magnesium concentration. Magnes Res. 1992;5:249-254.

93. Mahfouz MM, Zhou Q, Kummerow FA. Cholesterol oxides in plasma and lipoproteins of magnesium-deficient rabbits and effects of their lipoproteins on endothelial barrier function. Magnes Res. 1994;7:207-222.

94. Yokoyama S, Gu J, Kashima K, Nishida HI, Smith TL, Kummerow FA. Combined effects of magnesium deficiency and an atherogenic level of low density lipoprotein on uptake and metabolism of low density lipoprotein by cultured human endothelial cells. II. Electron microscopic data. Magnes Res. 1994;7:97-105.

95. Yokoyama S, Smith TL, Kawano KK, Kummerow FA. Effect of magnesium on secretion of platelet-derived growth factor by cultured human arterial smooth muscle cells. Magnes Res. 1996;9:93-99.

96. Zhou Q, Hulea S, Kummerow FA. The accentuating effect of low magnesium concentration on cholestane-3 beta, 5 alpha, 6 beta-triol-induced decrease of LDL uptake by cultured endothelial cells. Magnes Res. 1999;12:89-98.

97. Zhou Q, Kummerow FA. Modifying effect of 26-hydroxycholesterol on low- magnesium-induced atherosclerotic changes in the cultured human arterial smooth muscle cell. Magnes Res. 1993;6:121-126.

98. Zhou Q, Kummerow FA. The effects of magnesium deficiency on DNA and lipid synthesis in cultured human umbilical arterial endothelial cells. Magnes Res. 1995;8:145-150.

99. Zhou Q, Kummerow FA. Cholesterol metabolism in human umbilical arterial endothelial cells cultured in low magnesium media. Magnes Res. 1996;9:273-280.

100. Zhou Q, Mahfouz MM, Kummerow FA. Effect of dietary magnesium deficiency with/without cholesterol supplementation on phospholipid content in liver, plasma and erythrocytes of rabbits. Magnes Res. 1994;7:23-30.

101. Zhou Q, Olinescu RM, Kummerow FA. Influence of low magnesium concentrations in the medium on the antioxidant system in cultured human arterial endothelial cells. Magnes Res. 1999;12:19-29.

102. Zhou Q, Yuan C, Wei T, Kummerow FA. Effect of low magnesium concentration and cholestane-3beta, 5alpha, 6beta-triol on levels of LDL receptor in cultured fibroblasts. Magnes Res. 2002;15:3-10.

103. Sakuragi T, Kummerow FA. Antioxidative Activity of Derivatives off Vitamin B6 and activity and structurally related compounds. JAOCS. 1958;35:401-404.

104. Sakuragi T. The functions of vitamin B6 in Fat metabolism. JAOCS. 1959;36.

105. Kummerow FA, Olinescu RM, Fleischer L, Handler B, Shinkareva SV. The relationship of oxidized lipids to coronary artery stenosis. Atherosclerosis. 2000;149:181-190.

106. Lande KE, Sperry WM. Human atherosclerosis in relation to the cholesterol content of the blood serum. Arch Pathol. 1936;22:301-312.

107. Mann GV, Sperry A, Gray M, Jarashow D. Atherosclerosis in the Masai. Am J Epidemiol. 1972;95:26-37.

108. Goto Y. Lipid peroxides as a cause of vascular disease. In: Yagi K, ed. Lipid Peroxides in Biology and Medicine. New York: Academic Press; 1982:295-303.

109. Zhou Q, Jimi S, Smith TL, Kummerow FA. The effect of 25-hydroxycholesterol on accumulation of intracellular calcium. Cell Calcium. 1991;12:467-476.

110. Zhou Q, Smith TL, Kummerow FA. Cytotoxicity of oxysterols on cultured smooth muscle cells from human umbilical arteries. Proc Soc Exp Biol Med. 1993;202:75-80.

111. Hessler JR, Morel DW, Lewis LJ, Chisolm GM. Lipoprotein oxidation and lipoprotein-induced cytotoxicity. Arteriosclerosis. 1983;3:215-222.

112. Holvoet P, Stassen JM, Van Cleemput J, Collen D, Vanhaecke J. Oxidized low density lipoproteins in patients with transplant-associated coronary artery disease. Arterioscler Thromb Vasc Biol. 1998;18:100-107.

113. Mahfouz MM, Kummerow FA. Oxysterols and TBARS are among the LDL oxidation products which enhance thromboxane A2 synthesis by platelets. Prostaglandins Other Lipid Mediat. 1998;56:197-217.

114. Naito C, Kawamura M, Yamamoto Y. Lipid peroxides as the initiating factor of atherosclerosis. Ann N Y Acad Sci. 1993;676:27-45.

115. Negre-Salvayre A, Fitoussi G, Reaud V, Pieraggi MT, Thiers JC, Salvayre R. A delayed and sustained rise of cytosolic calcium is elicited by oxidized LDL in cultured bovine aortic endothelial cells. FEBS Lett. 1992;299:60-65.

116. Sato Y, Hotta N, Sakamoto N, Matsuoka S, Ohishi N, Yagi K. Lipid peroxide level in plasma of diabetic patients. Biochem Med. 1979;21:104-107.

117. Smith LL. Cholesterol Autoxidation. New York: Plenum Press; 1981.

118. Zhou Q, Wasowicz E, Handler B, Fleischer L, Kummerow FA. An excess concentration of oxysterols in the plasma is cytotoxic to cultured endothelial cells. Atherosclerosis. 2000;149:191-197.

119. Smith TL, Kummerow FA. Effect of dietary vitamin E on plasma lipids and atherogenesis in restricted ovulator chickens. Atherosclerosis. 1989;75:105-109.

120. Smith T, Toda T, Kummerow FA. Plasma lipid peroxidation in hyperlipidemic chickens. Atherosclerosis. 1985;57:119-122.

121. Smith TL, Kummerow FA. Induction of serum lipid peroxidation in chickens. Artery. 1986;14:30-34.

122. Toda T, Leszczynski D, McGibbon WH, Kummerow FA. Coronary arterial lesions in sexually mature non-layers, layers, and roosters. Virchows Arch A Pathol Anat Histol. 1980;388:123-135.

123. Toda T, Leszczynski D, Nishimori I, Kummerow F. Arterial lesions in restricted-ovulator chickens with endogenous hyperlipidemia. Avian Dis. 1981;25:162-178.

124. Toda T, Nishimori I, Kummerow FA. Animal Model of Atherosclerosis Experimental Atherosclerosis in the Chicken Animal Model. J Jpn Atheroscler Soc. 1984;11:755-761.

125. Tokuyasu K, Imai H, Taura S, Cho BH, Kummerow FA. Aortic lesions in nonlaying hens with endogenous hyperlipidemia. Arch Pathol Lab Med. 1980;104:41-45.

126. Toda T, Leszczynski D, Kummerow F. Angiotoxic effects of dietary 7-ketocholesterol in chick aorta. Paroi Arterielle. 1981;7:167-175.

127. Toda T, Toda Y, Cho BH, Kummerow FA. Ultrastructural changes in the comb and aorta of chicks fed excess testosterone. Atherosclerosis. 1984;51:47-57.

128. Navab M, Berliner JA, Watson AD, et al. The Yin and Yang of oxidation in the development of the fatty streak. A review based on the 1994 George Lyman Duff Memorial Lecture. Arterioscler Thromb Vasc Biol. 1996;16:831-842.

129. Heinecke JW. Oxidants and antioxidants in the pathogenesis of atherosclerosis: implications for the oxidized low density lipoprotein hypothesis. Atherosclerosis. 1998;141:1-15.

130. Zhou Q, Jimi S, Smith TL, Kummerow FA. The effect of cholesterol on the accumulation of intracellular calcium. Biochim Biophys Acta. 1991;1085:1-6.

131. Hulea SA, Smith TL, Wasowicz E, Kummerow FA. Bilirubin sensitized photooxidation of human plasma low density lipoprotein. Biochim Biophys Acta. 1996;1304:197-209.

132. Hulea SA, Wasowicz E, Kummerow FA. Inhibition of metal-catalyzed oxidation of low-density lipoprotein by free and albumin-bound bilirubin. Biochim Biophys Acta. 1995;1259:29-38.

133. Olinescu R, Alexandrescu R, Hulea SA, Kummerow FA. Tissue lipid peroxidation may be triggered by increased formation of bilirubin in vivo. Res Commun Chem Pathol Pharmacol. 1994;84:27-34.

134. Olinescu RM, Kummerow FA. Fibrinogen is as efficient antioxidant. J Nur Biochem. 2001;12:162-169.

135. Kummerow F, Cook L, Wasowicz E, Jellen H. Changes in the Phospholipid composition of the arterial cell can result in severe atherosclerotic lesions. Journal of Nutritional Biochemistry 2001;12:602-607.

136. Zhou Q, Kummerow FA. Effects of 27-hydroxycholesterol on cellular sphingomyelin synthesis and Ca++ content in cultured smooth muscle cells. Biomed Environ Sci 1997; 10: 369-376.

137. Zhou Q, Kummerow FA. Alterations of Ca++ Uptake and Lipid Content in Cultured Human Arterial Smooth Muscle Cells Treated with 26-Hydrocholesterol. Artery 1994. 21(4): 182-192

138. Javitt NB. 26-Hydroxycholesterol: synthesis, metabolism, and biologic activities. J Lipid Res 1990; 31: 1527-1533.

139. Deuel H. The Lipids-Their Chemistry and Biochemistry. New York: Interscience Publisher Inc.; 1955.

140. Chow CK. Fatty Acids in Food and Their Health Implications. New York: Marcel Dekker, Inc.; 1922.

141. Bailey AE. Industrial Oil and Fat Products. New York: Interscience Publisher Inc.; 1951.

142. Institute of Medicine National Academy of Science. Dietary Reference Intake Part 1. Washington D.C.; 2003.

143. Kunau WH, Holman RT. Polyunsaturated Fatty Acids. Champaign, Ill: AOCS; 1977.

144. Schwartz JI, Agrawal NG, Hartford AH, et al. The effect of etoricoxib on the pharmacodynamics and pharmacokinetics of warfarin. J Clin Pharmacol. 2007;47:620-627.

145. Ratageri VH, Shepur TA, Kiran G. Vitreous hemorrhage secondary to vitamin K deficiency bleeding. Indian J Pediatr. 2007;74:314.

146. Couzin J. Drug safety. Withdrawal of Vioxx casts a shadow over COX-2 inhibitors. Science. 2004;306:384-385.

147. Burr GO, Burr MM. On the Nature and Role of the Fatty Acids Essential in Nutrition. J Biol Chem. 1930;86:587.

148. Kummerow FA, Pan HP, Hickman H. The effect of dietary fat on the reproductive performance and the mixed fatty acid composition of fat-deficient rats. J Nutr. 1952;46:489-498.

149. Uauy R, Hoffman DR, Peirano P, Birch DG, Birch EE. Essential fatty acids in visual and brain development. Lipids. 2001;36:885-895.

150. Siegel G, al. e. Basic Neurochemistry. 4th ed. New York: Raven Press, Ltd.; 1989.

151. Innis SM. Essential fatty acids in growth and development. Prog Lipid Res. 1991;30:39-103.

152. Personal Communication: Dr. Toshiro Nishida Professor of Food Science and Nutrition at University of Illinois Urbana-Champaign, IL.

153. Pilgeram L. Atherogenesis and fibrinogen: historical perspective and current status. Naturwissenschaften. 1993;80:547-555.

154. Pilgeram L. Atherogenesis: Historical Perspective, biochemical mechanism, and current status. . Cardio Eng. 2003;2:111-12

155. Goldstein JL, Brown MS. Binding and degradation of low density lipoproteins by cultured human fibroblasts. Comparison of cells from a normal subject and from a patient with homozygous familial hypercholesterolemia. J Biol Chem. 1974;249:5153-5162.

156. Kummerow FA. Improving Hydrogenated Fat for the World Population. Prevention and Control. 2005;1:157-164.

157. Food labeling: trans fatty acids in nutrition labeling, nutrient content claims, and health claims. Final rule. Fed Regist. 2003;68:41433-41506.

158. Kummerow FA. The negative effects of Hydrogenated trans fats and what to do about them. Atherosclerosis. 2009;205:458-65.

159. Zalewski S, Kummerow FA. Rapeseed oil in a two-component margarine base stock. JAOCS. 1968;45:87-92.

160. Kummerow FA, Zhou Q, Mahfouz MM, Smiricky MR, Grieshop CM, Schaeffer DJ. Trans fatty acids in hydrogenated fat inhibited the synthesis of the polyunsaturated fatty acids in the phospholipid of arterial cells. Life Sci. 2004:74(22):2707-23.

161. Kummerow FA, Mahfouz M, Zhou Q, Masterjohn C. Effects of Trans Fats on Prostacyclin Production. Scandinavian Journal. Under review.

162. James AT, Martin AJ. Gas-liquid partition chromatography: the separation and micro-estimation of ammonia and the methylamines. Biochem J. 1952;52:238-242.

163. Meyer WH, Manager. Professional & Regulatory Relations, Proctor & Gamble Co. 1967.

164. Lawson LD, Kummerow FA. beta-Oxidation of the coenzyme A esters of elaidic, oleic, and stearic acids and their full-cycle intermediates by rat heart mitochondria. Biochim Biophys Acta. 1979;573:245-254.

165. Lawson LD, Kummerow FA. beta-Oxidation of the coenzyme A esters of vaccenic, elaidic, and petroselaidic acids by rat heart mitochondria. Lipids. 1979;14:501-503.

166. The National Diet-Heart Study Final Report. Circulation. 1968;37:I1-428.

167. Emken EA, Dutton HJ. Geometrical and Positional Fatty Acid Isomers. Champaign, IL: AOCS; 1979.

168. Mosley EE, Wright AL, McGuire MK, McGuire MA. trans fatty acids in milk produced by women in the United States. Am J Clin Nutr. 2005;82:1292-1297.

169. Stary HC, Chandler AB, Dinsmore RE, et al. A definition of advanced types of atherosclerotic lesions and a histological classification of atherosclerosis. A report from the Committee on Vascular Lesions of the Council on Arteriosclerosis, American Heart Association. Arterioscler Thromb Vasc Biol. 1995;15:1512-1531.

170. Kummerow FA, Zhou Q, Mahfouz MM, Effects of trans fatty acids on calcium influx into human arterial endothelial cells. Am. J. Clin. NUtr. 1999;70:832-838.

171. FDA. Questions and Answers about Trans Fat Nutrition Labeling. Washington D.C.: Office of Nutritional Products, Labeling and dietary Supplements; 2006.

172. Stender S, Dyerberg J, Hansen HS. First international symposium on trans fatty acids and health. Rugstedfaard, Rugested Kyst, Denmark, 11-13 September 2005. Atherosclerosis. 2006;7:2-10.

173. REF: http://www.cdc.gov/media/releases/2012/p0208_trans-fatty_acids.html accessed 9/12/13

174. Data supplied by Robert Anderson, chief statistician, Center for Disease Control and the National Center for Health Statistics

175. Moses C. Medical Director of the AHA. Dallas, TX: American Heart Association; 1968.

176. Courtesy of W.H. Meyer, Manager-Professional & Regulatory Relations at Procter & Gamble, 1968.

177. Death Rates for Disease of Heart, by Sex, Race, Hispanic Origin, and Age: United States, Selected Years 1950-2004. National Center for Health Statistics. Washington D.C.;2006

178. Staprans I, Pan XM, PRapp JH, Feingold KR. Oxidized cholesterol in the diet accelerates the development of aortic atherosclerosis in cholesterol-fed rabbits. Arterioscler. Thromb. Vas. Biol. 1998;18:977-983.

179. Johnson OC, Sakuragi T, Kummerow FA. A Comparitive Study of the Nutritive Value of Thermally Oxidized Oils. J Am Oil Chem Soc. 1956;33:433-435.

180. Bhalerao VR, Johnson OC, Kummerow FA. Effect of Thermal Oxidative Polymerization on the Growth-Promoting Value of Some Fractions of Butterfat. J. Dairy Sci. 1959;42:1057-1062.

181. Hemans C, Kummerow F, Perkins EG. Influence of protein and vitamin levels on the nutritional value of heated fats for rats. J Nutr. 1973;103:1665-1672.

182. Witting LA, Nishida T, Johnson OC, Kummerow FA. The Relationship of Pyridoxine and Riboflavin to the Nutritional Value of Polymerized Fats. J Am Oil Chem Soc. 1957;34:421-424.

183. Roffo AH. Carcinogenic Value of Oxidated Oils; Sunflower Oil. Am J Digest. 1946;13:33-38.

184. Sugai M, Witting LA, Tsuchiyama H, Kummerow FA. The effect of heated fat on the carcinogenic activity of 2-acetylaminofluorene. Cancer Res. 1962;22:510-519.

185. Frankel EN. Lipid Oxidation. Davis, California: The Oily Press, University of California; 2005.

186. Peng S, Mortin RJ. Biological Effects of Cholesterol Oxides: CRC Press; 1992.

187. USDA Nutrient Data Laboratory, Washington D.C.; 2005.

188. Rose WC, Wixom RL, Lockhart HB, Lambert GF. The amino acid requirements of man. XV. The valine requirement; summary and final observations. J Biol Chem. 1955;217:987-995.

189. Recommended Dietary Allowance. Food and Nutrition Board. 18th rev. ed. ed. Washington D.C.: National Academy of Sciences; 1974.

190. Cuaron JA, Chapple RP, Easter RA. Nitrogen metabolism of gravid and nongravid female swine fed every third day. J Anim Sci. 1983;56:96-100.

191. Kokatnur MG, Kummerow FA. Amino acid imbalance and cholesterol levels in chicks. J Nutr. 1961;75:319-329.

192. Greene CM, Zern TL, Wood RJ, et al. Maintenance of the LDL cholesterol:HDL cholesterol ratio in an elderly population given a dietary cholesterol challenge. J Nutr. 2005;135:2793-2798.

193. Herron KL, Fernandez ML. Are the current dietary guidelines regarding egg consumption appropriate? J Nutr. 2004;134:187-190.

194. Knopp RH, Retzlaff BM, Walden CE, et al. A double-blind, randomized, controlled trial of the effects of two eggs per day in moderately hypercholesterolemic and combined hyperlipidemic subjects taught the NCEP step I diet. J Am Coll Nutr. 1997;16:551-561.

195. Vorster HH, Benade AJ, Barnard HC, et al. Egg intake does not change plasma lipoprotein and coagulation profiles. Am J Clin Nutr. 1992;55:400-410.

196. Hu FB, Stampfer MJ, Rimm EB, et al. A prospective study of egg consumption and risk of cardiovascular disease in men and women. JAMA. 1999;281:1387-1394.

197. Flynn MA, Nolph GB, Flynn TC, Kahrs R, Krause G. Effect of dietary egg on human serum cholesterol and triglycerides. Am J Clin Nutr. 1979;32:1051-1057.

198. Dawber TR, Nickerson RJ, Brand FN, Pool J. Eggs, serum cholesterol, and coronary heart disease. Am J Clin Nutr. 1982;36:617-625.

199. Katz DL, Evans MA, Nawaz H, et al. Egg consumption and endothelial function: a randomized controlled crossover trial. Int J Cardiol. 2005;99:65-70.

200. Kummerow FA, Kim Y, Hull J, et al. The influence of egg consumption on the serum cholesterol level in human subjects. Am J Clin Nutr. 1977;30:664-673.

201. Messinger WJ, Porosowska Y, Steele JM. Effect of feeding egg yolk and cholesterol on serum cholesterol levels. Arch Med Interna. 1950;86:189-195.

202. Kummerow FA. Official Transcript of Proceedings at National Commission on Egg Nutrition. Washington D.C.: Federal Trade Commission; June 12, 1975.

203. Kummerow FA. Official Transcripts of Testimony Federal Trade Commission Chicago, IL; 1976.

204. Watson R. Eggs and Health Promotion. Ames, Iowa: Iowa State Press; 2002.

205. Lappe FM. Diet for a Small Planet. New York, NY: Ballantine Books; 1971.

206. Nestle M. What to Eat: An aisle by aisle guide to savvy food choices and good eating: Farrar Straus and Giroux; 2006.

207. USDA's Annual Fall Crop Summary, Winter Wheat Seedings, and Grain Stocks Report. Illinois: Illinois Department of Agriculture; January 12, 2007.

208. Navidi MK, Kummerow FA. Nutritional value of Egg Beaters compared with "farm fresh eggs". Pediatrics. 1974;53:565-566.

209. Kummerow FA. Optimum nutrition through better planning of world agriculture. World Rev Nutr Diet. 1985;45:1-41.

210. CIA. The CIA's World Factbook; April 25, 2007.

211. http://www.fas.usda.gov/psdonline/circulars/livestock_poultry.pdf, April 2013, accessed September 11, 2013 The SOYBEAN REference is http://legroupindustries.com/top-10-exporters-of-soybeans-and-soybean-meals-by-country/ July 2013 also accessed on 9/11/2013

212. Rand NT, Scott HM, Kummerow FA. Dietary Fat in the Nutrition of the Growing Chick. Poult Sci. 1958;37:1075-1085.

213. Kummerow FA, Ueno A, Nishida T, Kokatnur M. Unsaturated Fatty Acids and Plasma Lipids. Am J Clin Nutr. 1960;8:62-67.

214. Beer MK. The Merck Manual of Medical Information. 2nd Home ed. White House Sta, NJ: Merck Research Laboratories; 2013.

215. http://www.ers.usda.gov/data-products/sugar-and-sweeteners-yearbook-tables.aspx#25512 accessed 9/11/13

216. Buzby J, Farah H. U.S. Food Consumption up 16 Percent since 1970 Amber Waves. Vol 3; 2005.

217. By The Numbers: What Americans Drink In a Year. Huffington Post. (2011). http://www.huffingtonpost.com/2011/06/27/americans-soda-beer_n_885340.html?view=print&comm_ref=false.

218. Dhingra R, Sullivan L, Jacques P, et al. Soft Drink Consumption and Risk of Developing Cardiometabolic Risk Factors and the Metabolic Syndrome in Middle-Aged Adults in the Community. Circulation. 2007;116:480-488.

219. http://www.mayoclinic.com/health/artificial-sweeteners/MY00073

220. Harnack L, Stang J, Story M. Soft drink consumption among US children and adolescents: nutritional consequences. J Am Diet Assoc. 1999;99:436-441.

221. Margolskee RF, Dyer J, Kokrashvili Z, et al. T1R3 and gustducin in gut sense sugars to regulate expression of Na+ - glucose cotransporter 1. PNAS. 2007;10:1-6.

222. http://www.ncbi.nlm.nih.gov/pmc/articles/PMC3220878/ accessed 9/11/13

223. Montana Wheat and Barley Committee. Wheat Kernel. Great Falls, Montana; 2001.

224. Fleming SE, O'Donnell AU, Perman JA. Influence of frequent and long-term bean consumption on colonic function and fermentation. Am J Clin Nutr. 1985;41:909-918.

225. http://www.ers.usda.gov/media/866543/cornusetable.html, accessed 9/12/13

226. Fiber, Total Dietary Content of Selected Foods per Common Measure: USDA National Nutrient Database; 2002.

227. Lanza E, Jones DY, Block G, Kessler L. Dietary fiber intake in the US population. Am J Clin Nutr. 1987;46:790-797.

228. Newman HA, Kummerow FA, Scott HM. Dietary Saponin, A Factor Which May Reduce Liver and Serum Cholesterol Levels. Poult Sci. 1958;37:42-46.

229. Potter GC, Kummerow FA. Chemical similarity and biological activity of the saponins isolated from alfalfa and soy-beans. Science. 1954;120:224-225.

230. Bjorck I, Elmstahl HL. The glycaemic index: importance of dietary fibre and other food properties. Proc Nutr Soc. 2003;62:201-206.

231. Tucker KL. Dietary Intake and Coronary Heart Disease: A Variety of Nutrients and Phytochemicals Are Important. Curr Treat Options Cardiovasc Med. 2004;6:291-302.

232. Anderson JW. Whole grains protect against atherosclerotic cardiovascular disease. Proc Nutr Soc. 2003;62:135-142.

233. Singh RB, Mori H, Kummerow FA. Macro and Trace Mineral Metabolism in Coronary Heart Disease. Trace Elements in Medicine. 1992;3:144-156.

234. Calcium Ca Content of Selected Foods per Common Measure: USDA National Nutrient Database; 2002.

235. DiPette DJ, Greilich PE, Nickols GA, et al. Effect of dietary calcium supplementation on blood pressure and calciotropic hormones in mineralocorticoid-salt hypertension. J Hypertens. 1990;8:515-520.

236. Elwood PC, Sweetnam PM, Beasley WH, Jones D, France R. Magnesium and calcium in the myocardium: cause of death and area differences. Lancet. 1980;2:720-722.

237. Potassium K Content of Selected Foods per Common Measure: USDA National Nutrient Database; 2002.

201

238. Altura BM, Altura BT. New perspectives on the role of magnesium in the pathophysiology of the cardiovascular system. II. Experimental aspects. Magnesium. 1985;4:245-271.

239. Seelig MS. Magnesium Deficiency in Pathogenesis of Disease. New York, NY: Plenum Publishing Corp.; 1980.

240. Seelig MS, Heggtveit HA. Magnesium interrelationships in ischemic heart disease: a review. Am J Clin Nutr. 1974;27:59-79.

241. Magnesium Content of Selected Foods per Common Measure: USDA National Nutrient Database; 2002. 175

242. Singh NK, Mori H, Kokatnur M, Kummerow FA. Nutrition in Coronary Heart Disease and Sudden Cardiac Death. Moradabad, India: International College of Nutrition; 1991.

243. Bostrom H, Wester PO. Trace elements in drinking water and death rate in cardiovascular disease. Acta Med Scand. 1967;181:465-473.

244. Schroeder HA, Kraemer LA. Cardiovascular mortality, municipal water, and corrosion. Arch Environ Health. 1974;28:303-311.

245. Crawford T, Crawford MD. Prevalence and pathological changes of ischaemic heart-disease in a hard-water and in a soft-water area. Lancet. 1967;1:229-232.

246. Klevay LM. The Role of Copper, Zinc and Other Chemical Elements in Ischemis Heart Disease. In: Renner OM, Chan WY, eds. Metabolism of Trace Metals in Man. Vol 1. Boca Raton, FL: CRC Press; 1984.

247. Kromhout D, Wibowo AA, Herber RF, et al. Trace metals and coronary heart disease risk indicators in 152 elderly men (the Zutphen Study). Am J Epidemiol. 1985;122:378-385.

248. O'Dell BL. Biochemistry of copper. Med Clin North Am. 1976;60:687-703.

249. Tiber AM, Sakhaii M, Joffe CD, Ratnaparkhi MV. Relative value of plasma copper, zinc, lipids and lipoproteins as markers for coronary artery disease. Atherosclerosis. 1986;62:105-110.

250. Uusitupa MI, Kumpulainen JT, Voutilainen E, et al. Effect of inorganic chromium supplementation on glucose tolerance, insulin response, and serum lipids in noninsulin-dependent diabetics. Am J Clin Nutr. 1983;38:404-410.

251. Newman HA, Leighton RF, Lanese RR, Freedland NA. Serum chromium and angiographically determined coronary artery disease. Clin Chem. 1978;24:541-544.

252. Narsigna Rao BS, Deoschale TG, Pant KC. Nutrient Composition of Indian Foods. Hyderabad, India: National Institute of Nutrition Publication; 1989.

253. Tipton IH, Schroeder HA, Perry HM, Jr., Cook MJ. Trace Elements in Human Tissue. 3. Subjects from Africa, the near and Far East and Europe. Health Phys. 1965;11:403-451.

254. Shamberger RJ. Selenium and heart disease II. Selenium and other trance metal intakes and hear disease in 25 countries Trace Substance in Environmental Health. 1978;2:48.

255. Jiang Y. Influence of barium and selenium on explanted heart cells 3rd int Symp on selenium in Biol and Med. Beijing. China; 1984.

256. Kris-Etherton PM, Lichtenstein AH, Howard BV, Steinberg D, Witztum JL. Antioxidant vitamin supplements and cardiovascular disease. Circulation. 2004;110:637-641.

257. Handelman GJ. Vitamin Facts. . University of Mass. Lowell; 2005.

258. Gopalan C. Vitamin A deficiency and childhood mortality. Lancet. 1992;340:177-178. 176

259. Berry RJ, Li Z, Erickson JD, et al. Prevention of neural-tube defects with folic acid in China. China-U.S. Collaborative Project for Neural Tube Defect Prevention. N Engl J Med. 1999;341:1485-1490.

260. Lonn E, Yusuf S, Arnold MJ, et al. Homocysteine lowering with folic acid and B vitamins in vascular disease. N Engl J Med. 2006;354:1567-1577.

261. Woo KS, Chook P, Lolin YI, et al. Hyperhomocyst(e)inemia is a risk factor for arterial endothelial dysfunction in humans. Circulation. 1997;96:2542-2544.

262. Clarke R, Lewington S, Donald A, et al. Underestimation of the importance of homocysteine as a risk factor for cardiovascular disease in epidemiological studies. J Cardiovasc Risk. 2001;8:363-369.

263. Shimakawa T, Nieto FJ, Malinow MR, Chambless LE, Schreiner PJ, Szklo M. Vitamin intake: a possible determinant of plasma homocyst(e)ine among middle-aged adults. Ann Epidemiol. 1997;7:285-293.

264. Szamosi T, Roth E, Szamosi T, Jr., Tomsits E, Tordai A, Szabo T. Hyperhomocysteinemia, enzyme polymorphism and thiobarbituric Acid reactive system in children with high coronary risk family history. J Am Coll Nutr. 2004;23:386-390.

265. Malinow MR, Sexton G, Averbuch M, Grossman M, Wilson D, Upson B. Homocysteine in daily practice: levels in coronary artery disease. Coronary Arter Dis. 1990;1:215-220.

266. Holmes RP, Kummerow FA. The relationship of adequate and excessive intake of vitamin D to health and disease. J Am Coll Nutr. 1983;2:173-199.

267. MacLaughlin JA, Anderson RR, Holick MF. Spectral character of sunlight modulates photosynthesis of previtamin D3 and its photoisomers in human skin. Science. 1982;216:1001-1003.

268. Dale AE, Lowenberg ME. Consumption of vitamin D in fortified and natural foods and in vitamin preparations. J Pediatr. 1967;70:952-955.

269. Hass GM, Trueheart RE, Taylor CB, Stumpe M. An experimental histologic study of hypervitaminosis D. Am J Pathol. 1958;34:395-431.

270. Mundy GR, Raisz LG. Disorders of bone resorption. In: Bronner F, Coburn JW, eds. Disorder of Mineral Metabolism. Vol III. New York: Academic Press; 1981:1-66.

271. Greer FR, Searcy JE, Levin RS, Steichen JJ, Steichen-Asche PS, Tsang RC. Bone mineral content and serum 25-hydroxyvitamin D concentrations in breast-fed infants with and without supplemental vitamin D: one-year follow- up. J Pediatr. 1982;100:919-922.

272. Hollis BW, Wagner CL. Assessment of dietary vitamin D requirements during pregnancy and lactation. Am J Clin Nutr. 2004;79:717-726.

273. U.S. International Trade commission Publication 920: Synthetic organic chemicals. In: U.S. Production and Sales, ed.; 1977, 1978. 177

274. Steenbock H. The induction of growth promoting and calcifying properties in a ration by exposure to light. Science. 1924;60:224-225.

275. Food and Nutrition board, National Academy of Sciences: Recommended dietary allowances. In: Sciences Office of Publications, ed. Washington: Committee of Dietary Allowances; 1980.

276. Seelig MS. Are American children still getting an excess of vitamin D? Hyperreactive children at risk. Clin Pediatr (Phila). 1970;9:380-383.

277. Taylor WH. Renal calculi and self-medication with multivitamin preparations containing vitamin D. Clin Sci. 1972;42:515-522.

278. Kummerow FA, Cho BH, Huang WY, et al. Additive risk factors in atherosclerosis. Am J Clin Nutr. 1976;29:579-584.

279. Dietary Supplement Fact Sheet: Vitamin D: National Institute of Health Office of Dietary Supplements. ; 2005.

280. Brown BG, Cheung MC, Lee AC, Zhao XQ, Chait A. Antioxidant vitamins and lipid therapy: end of a long romance? Arterioscler Thromb Vasc Biol. 2002;22:1535-1546.

281. Steinberg D, Witztum JL. Is the oxidative modification hypothesis relevant to human atherosclerosis? Do the antioxidant trials conducted to date refute the hypothesis? Circulation. 2002;105:2107-2111.

282. Mahfouz MM, Kummerow FA. Vitamin C or Vitamin B6 supplementation prevent the oxidative stress and decrease of prostacyclin generation in homocysteinemic rats. Int J Biochem Cell Biol. 2004;36:1919-1932.

283. Markham KR, Anderson OM. Flavonoids: Chemistry, Biochemistry, and Applications. Boca Raton, FL: Taylor and Francis; 2006.

284. Handelman GJ, Nightingale ZD, Lichtenstein AH, Schaefer EJ, Blumberg JB. Lutein and zeaxanthin concentrations in plasma after dietary supplementation with egg yolk. Am J Clin Nutr. 1999;70:247-251.

285. Hu FB. Plant-based foods and prevention of cardiovascular disease: an overview. Am J Clin Nutr. 2003;78:544S-551S.

286. Nishino H, Murakosh M, Ii T, et al. Carotenoids in cancer chemoprevention. Cancer Metastasis Rev. 2002;21:257-264.

287. USDA. Choose My Plate. Washington D.C: United State Department of Agriculture; 2013.

288. Dimler RJ, Harris RS, Von Lowseci H. Wheat: Nutritional Evaluation of Food Processing. New York: John Wiley and Sons; 1960.

289. Fellers DA, al. e. Mechanical Debranning of Whole-Kernel Wheat. Composition, cooking characteristics and storage stability. Cereal Chemists. 1976;53:308.

290. Ingelett GE. Wheat: Production and Utilization. Vol 193. Westport, Conn.: Avi Publishing Co.; 1974. 178

291. Kent NL. Technology of Cereals with Special Reference to Wheat. Oxford, New York: Pergamon Press; 1975.

Index

A

Acute phase proteins, 36

Albumin, 11, 12, 35, 50

Aleurone, 110

American Heart Association, 18, 57, 58, 91, 179, 182

Amino acids

  building blocks, 66, 72, 157

  essential, 12, 45, 61, 65, 67, 68, 69, 72, 73, 74, 76, 77, 78, 79, 80, 81, 83, 84, 87, 88, 92, 94, 98, 99, 100, 103, 104, 111, 142, 155, 157, 163, 164, 169

  oxidation, 35, 36, 123, 149, 150

Animal feeding studies, 100, 147

Anitchkow, Nikolaj, 15

Anitschkow, Nikolaj, 15

Antioxidants

  and coronary heart disease, 123, 151

  in diet, 123, 150, 151

Aorta, 14, 31, 187, 188

Apoprotein, 72

Arachidonic acid, 46, 48, 55, 56

Army Medical Corps, 16

Arterial calls, 15, 30, 31, 32

Arteries, 9, 11, 12, 13, 14, 15, 16, 17, 18, 29, 30, 31, 32, 35, 36, 37, 38, 49, 55, 56, 65, 87, 140, 144, 147, 157, 167, 174, 177

Artificial sweeteners, 108

Aspartame, 107

Atherosclerosis, 178

  and cholesterol, dietary, 8, 15, 22, 90

  animal models, 15, 16, 30, 87, 90

  development of, 30, 33, 35, 36, 140, 150

  risk factors, 14, 16, 29, 30, 32, 35, 140, 150, 157, 167

Atherosclerosis, International Society for, 179

Autopsies, 32

B

Bacteria, 5, 12, 121

Beriberi, 157

Beta blockers, 131

Branching segments, 31

Brassinosteroid, 9

Building blocks, 7, 11, 12, 65, 66, 72, 157

C

Calcification, 36, 147

Calcified deposit, 37

Calcium

and heart disease, 14, 37, 38, 82, 140, 145, 147

benefits of, 82, 124, 131, 145, 147

sources of, 9, 82, 120, 123, 131, 134, 136, 154

supplementation of, 82, 110, 145, 159

Calorie, 18, 49, 107, 119

Carbohydrates

in diet, 4, 45, 49, 66, 105, 106, 109, 111, 113, 114, 163, 165, 166, 168

Cardiovascular disease. *See* Coronary heart disease

Carotenoids, 41, 149, 151

Catheterization, 27, 179

Cell membranes, 36, 125

Cellulose, 117

CHD. *See* Coronary heart disease

Chevreul, Michel, 10

Chloride, 127

Chlorine, 26

Cholesterine, 10

Cholesterol, 176, 177

absorption, 16, 21, 22, 23, 51, 57, 65, 115, 117, 120, 136, 153

and atherosclerosis, 22, 33, 39, 90, 143

and coronary heart disease, 22, 33, 39, 90, 143

auto-oxidation of, 34

derivative, 39

hypothesis, 15, 23, 35

in eggs, 89

levels of, 18, 19, 20, 21, 22, 23, 27, 32, 33, 35, 36, 39, 55, 56, 95, 143

lowering drug, 25, 26, 27, 29, 39

metabolism, 22, 51, 115, 117, 153

negative perceptions of, 7, 8, 19, 33

synthesis of, 21, 22, 23, 33, 34, 36, 154

Cholestyramine, 25

Chromatography, 54, 58

208

211

Y

Z